ENDOCRINOLOGY

for kids

Medical School
FOR KIDS™

First paperback edition August 2022

Book design by Betty Nguyen & Brandon Pham

ISBN 978-1-957557-07-6 (paperback)

Printed in the United States of America

Published by Black Phoenix Press

www.mdforkids.org

To the friends and family who have supported and loved us unconditionally, and to the mentors who have guided and taught us more than we could have imagined:

Thank you.

Betty & Brandon

Medical School FOR KIDS™

Endocrinology

(en-doh-krih-NAA-luh-jee)

the branch of medicine concerned with the study and treatment of disorders of endocrine glands and hormones

Medical School FOR KIDS™

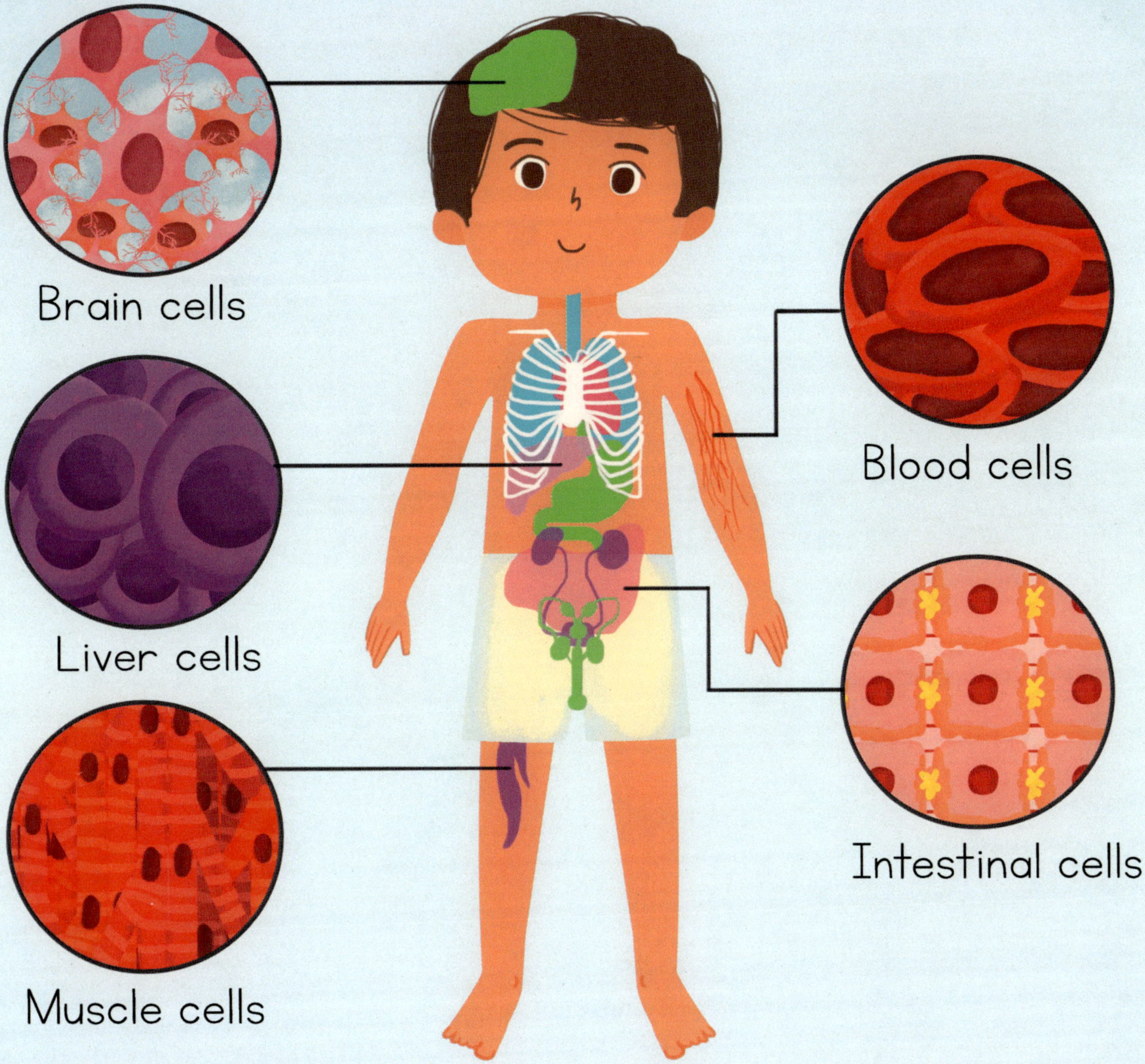

Cells are the basic building blocks of all living things. Our body is made up of *trillions* of cells!

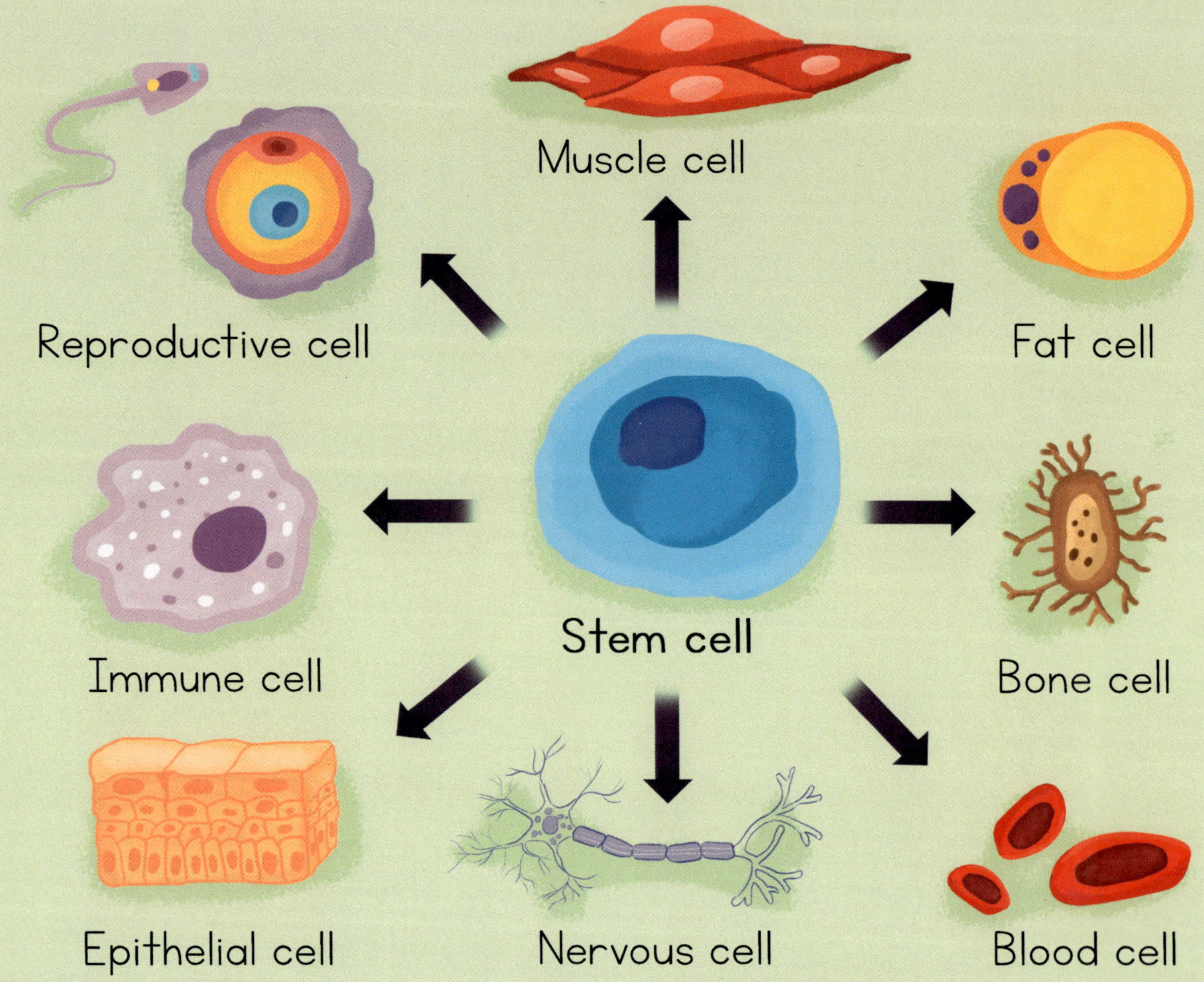

There are many types of cells in our body, and they each have different jobs. But how do our cells know which jobs to do?

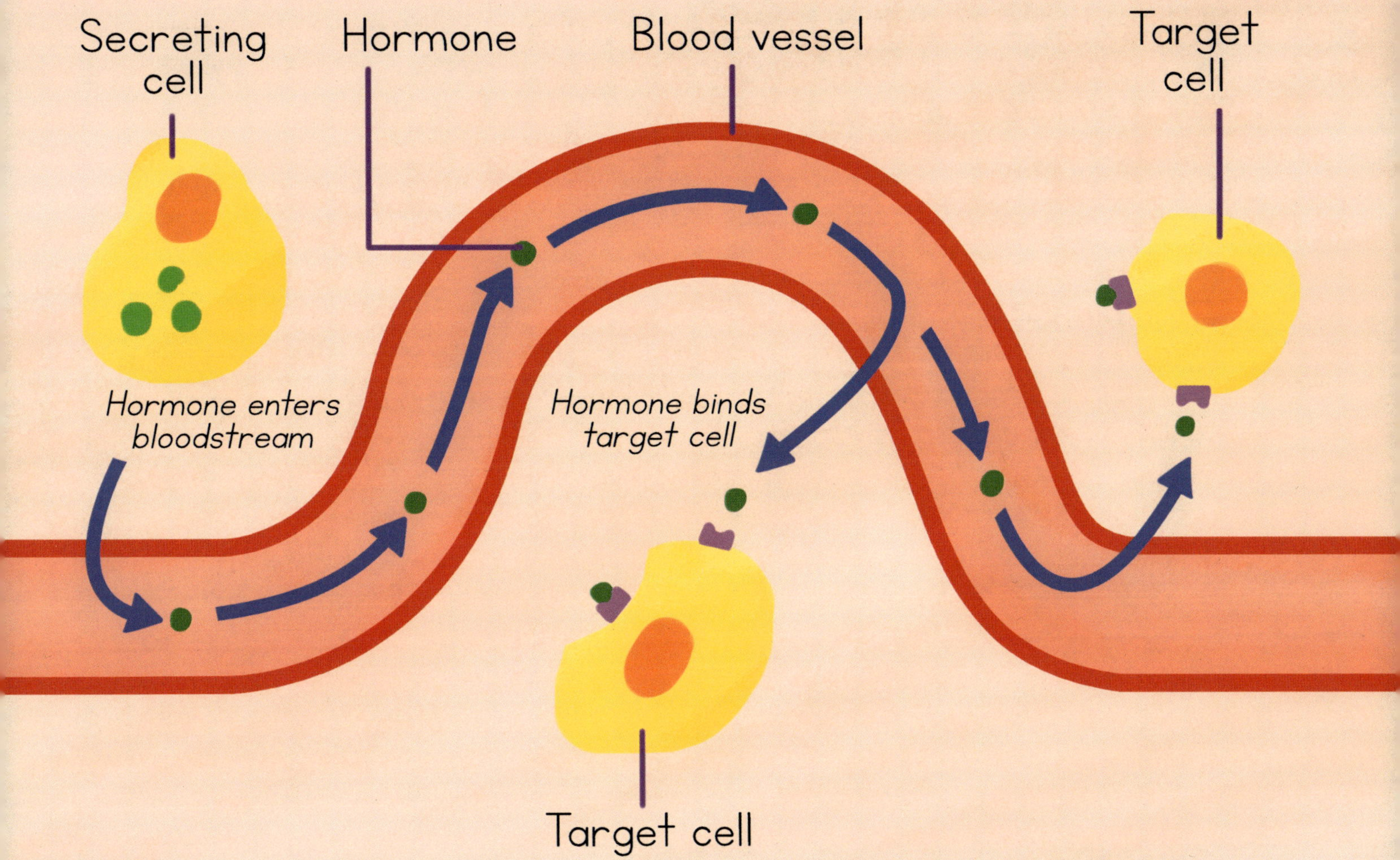

A **hormone** is a chemical made by our body that travels through our bloodstream to send messages to our cells.

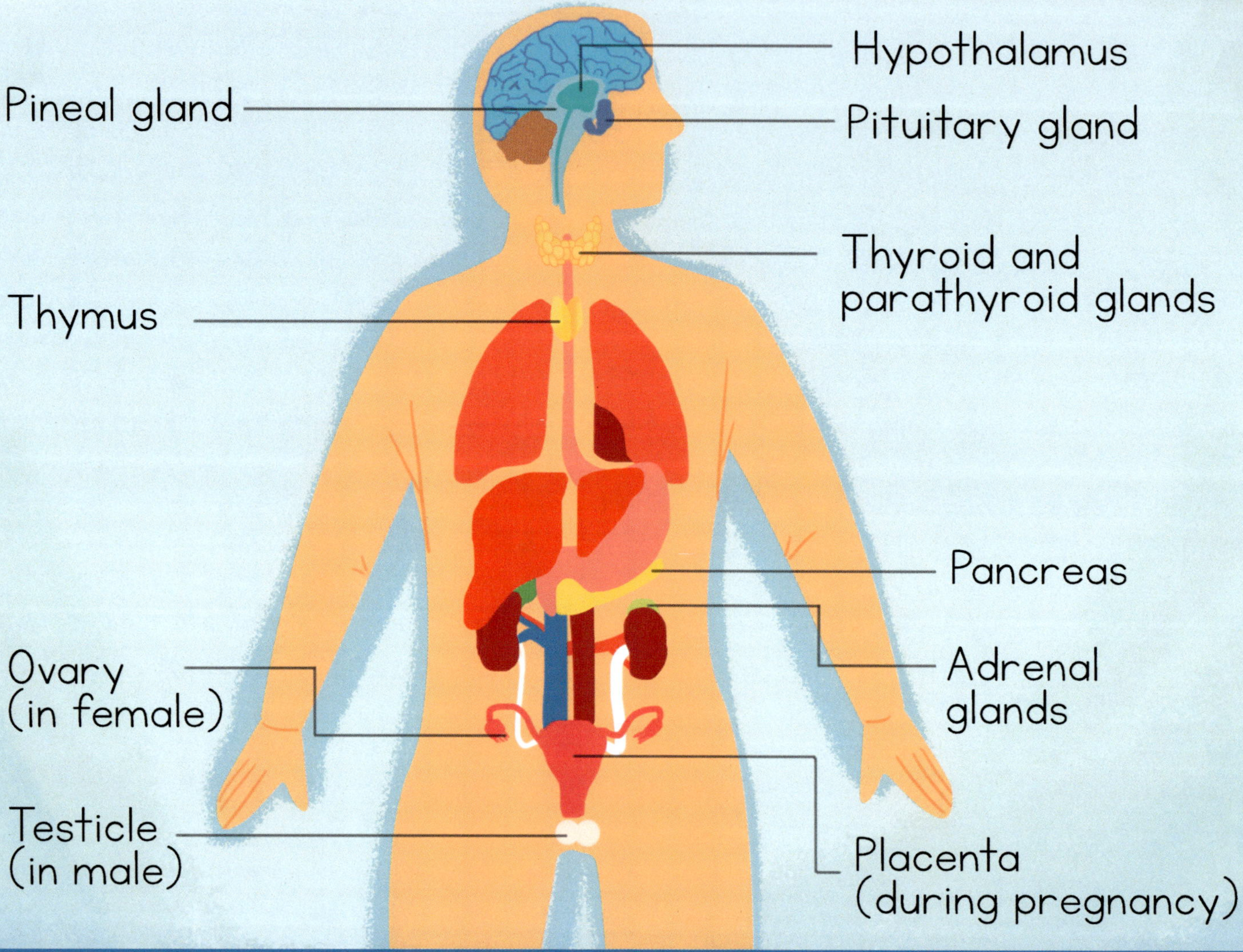

Hormones are made in specific places in our body called **endocrine glands**.

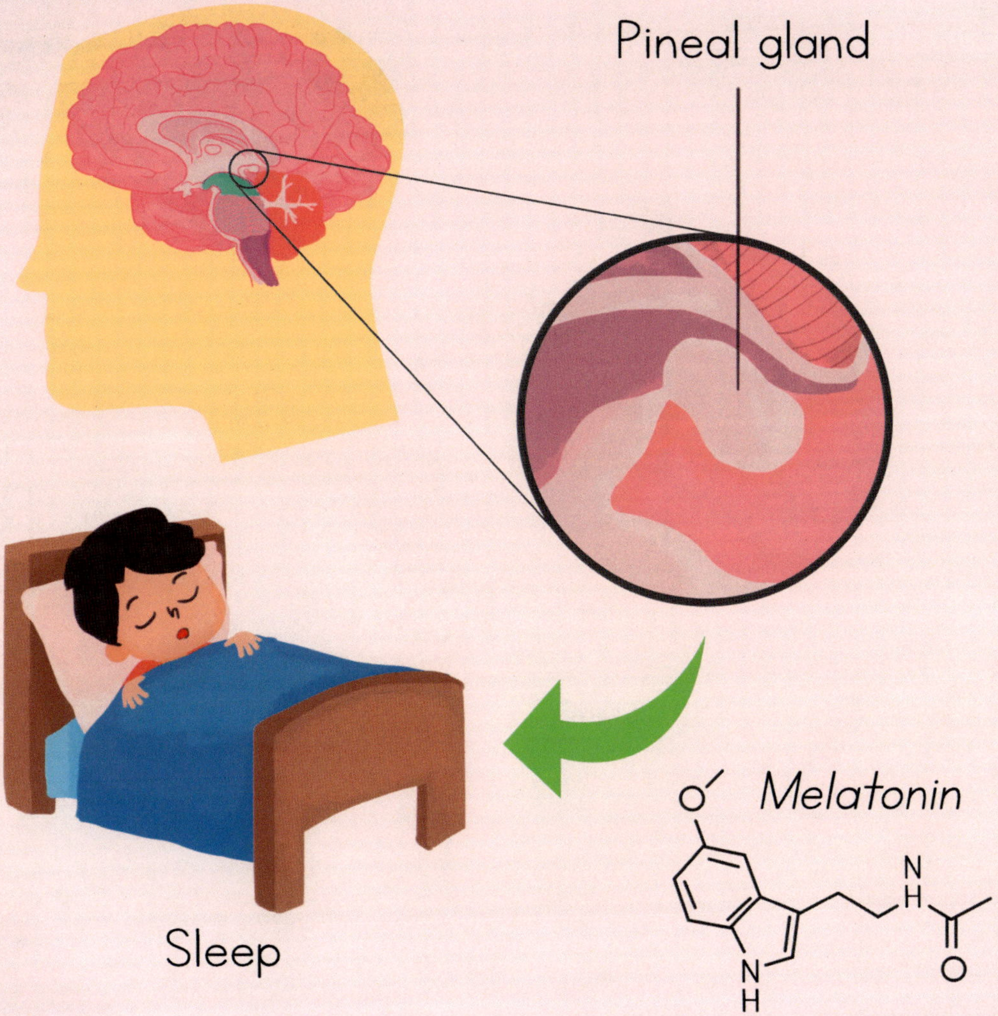

The **pineal gland** is a pea-sized gland in our brain that produces **melatonin**, a hormone that makes us sleepy when it's time to go to sleep.

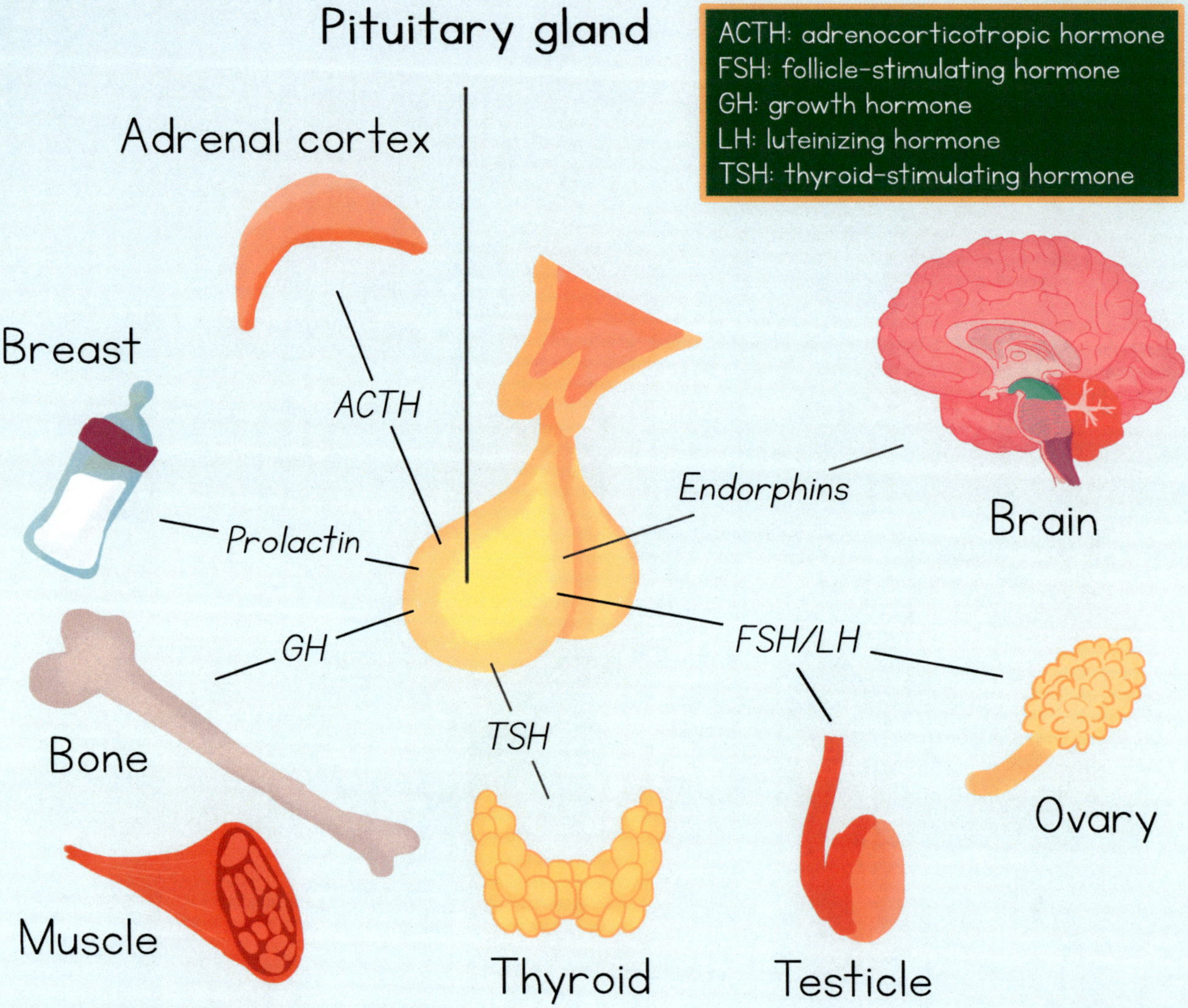

The **pituitary gland** is another pea-sized gland in our brain that produces hormones that control the activity of other organs and glands.

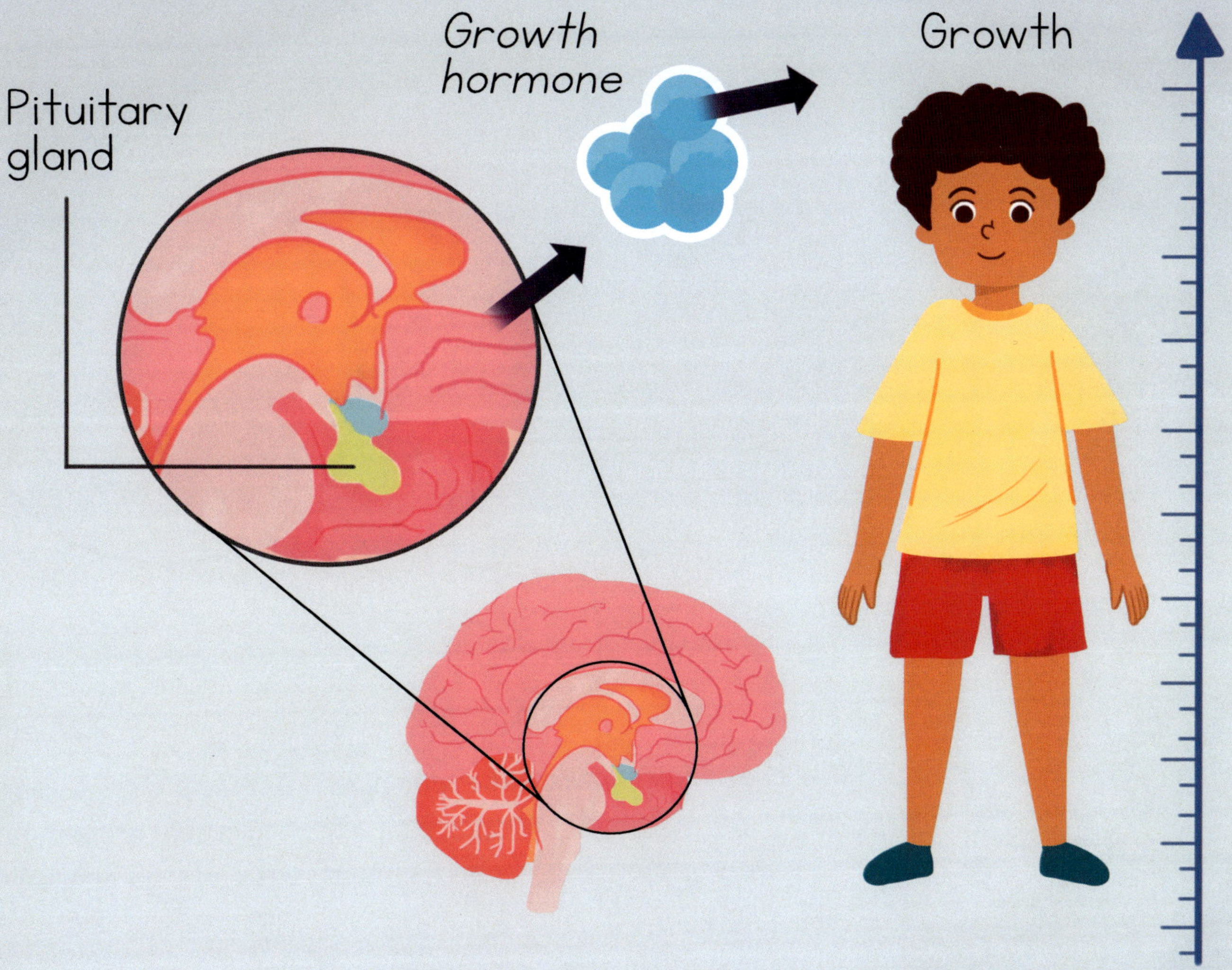

One example of a hormone made by the pituitary gland is **growth hormone**, which helps our body grow big and tall.

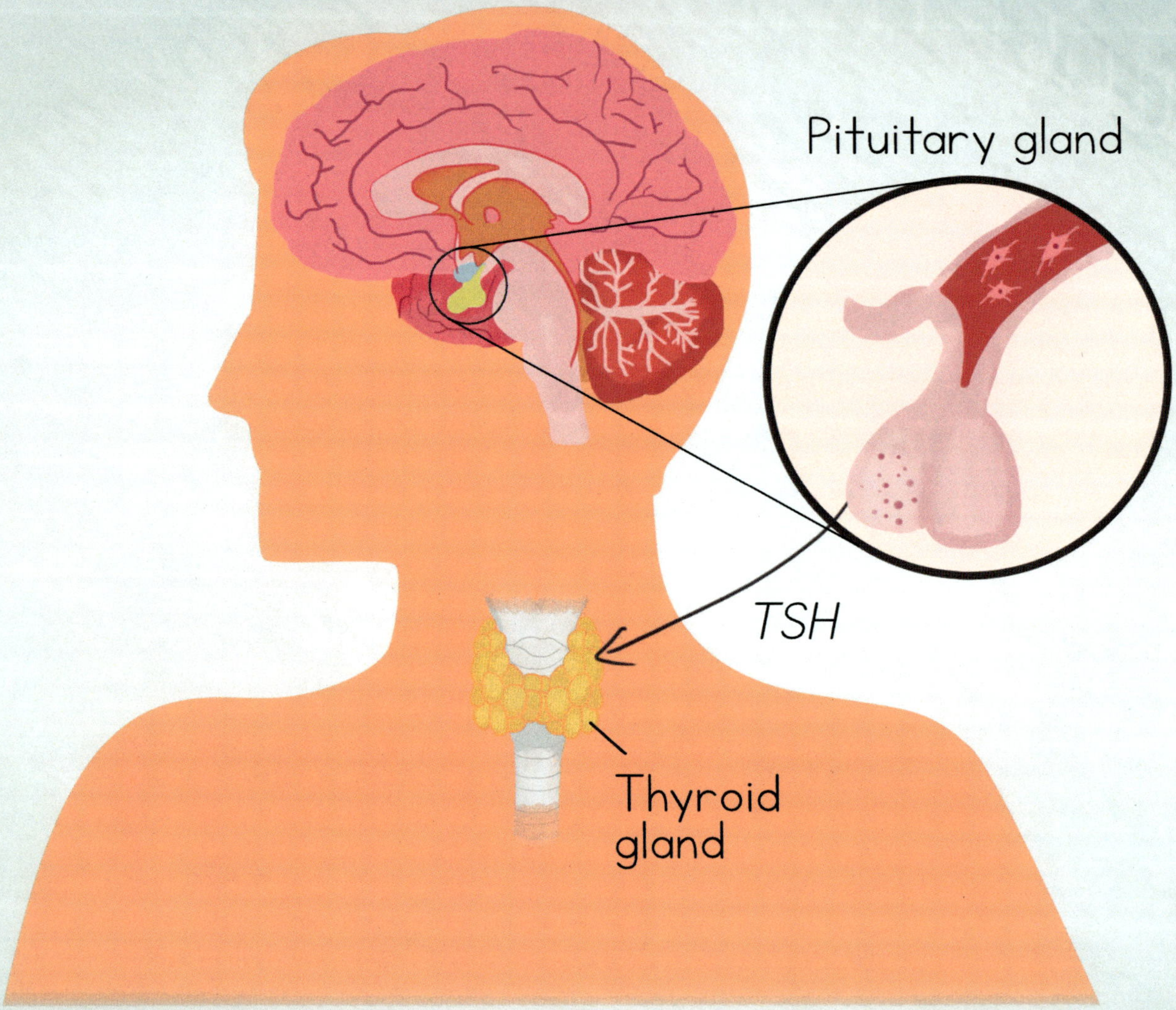

The pituitary gland also makes another hormone called **thyroid-stimulating hormone (TSH)**, which controls the activity of the **thyroid gland**.

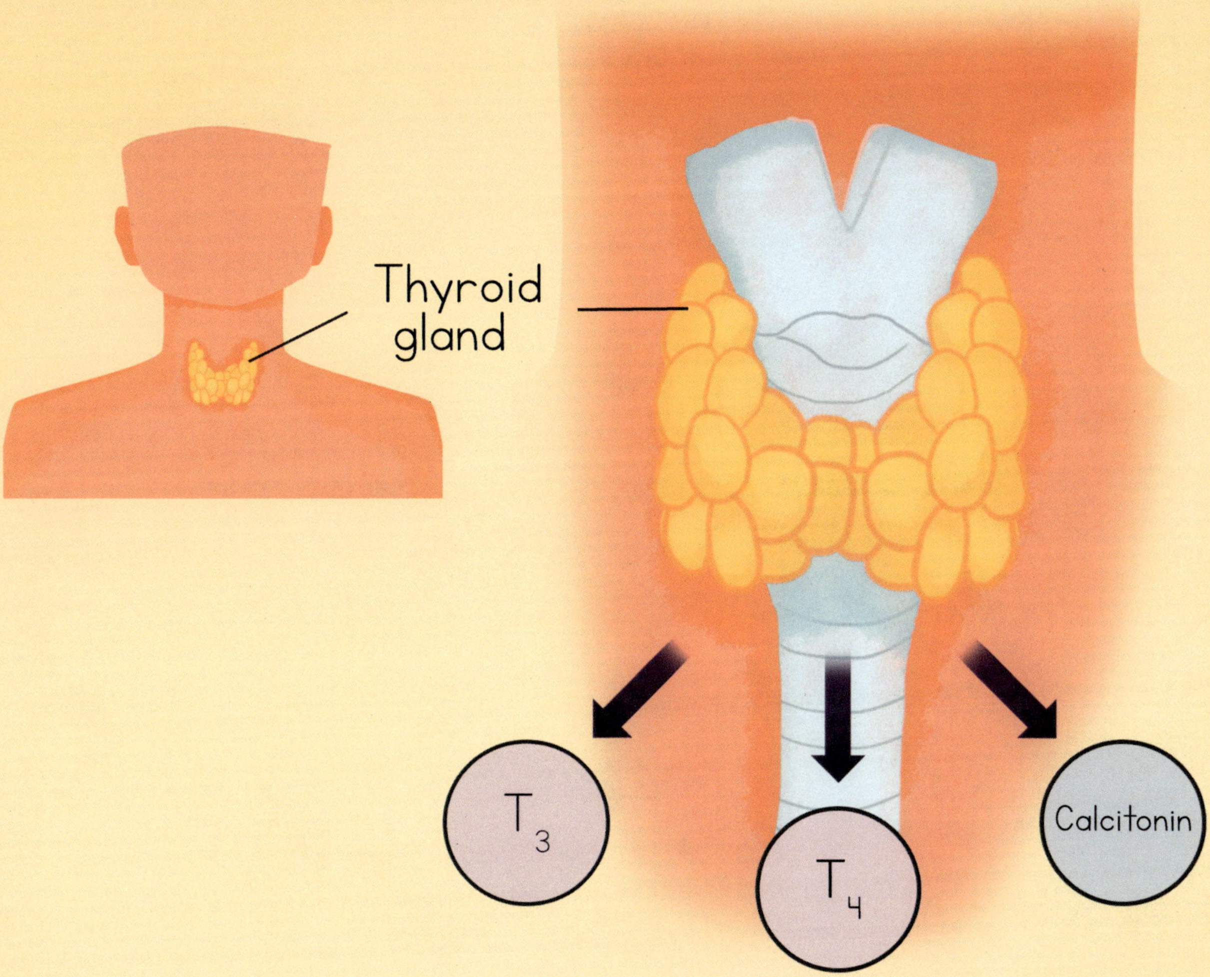

The **thyroid gland** is a butterfly-shaped gland in our neck that produces **thyroid hormone** (called **T3** and **T4**) and another hormone called **calcitonin**.

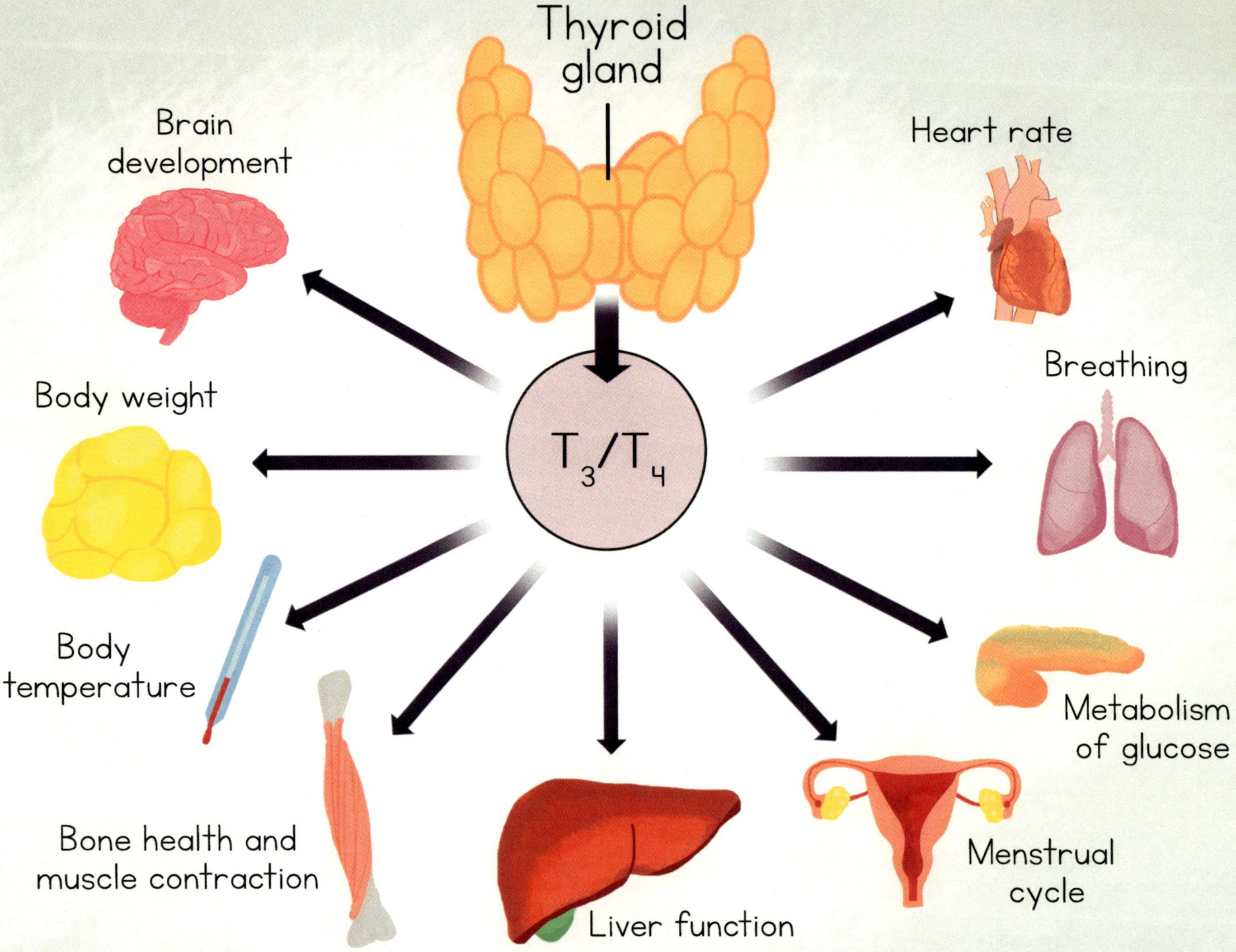

Thyroid hormone controls many important body functions, including how fast your cells burn fuels from food to make energy.

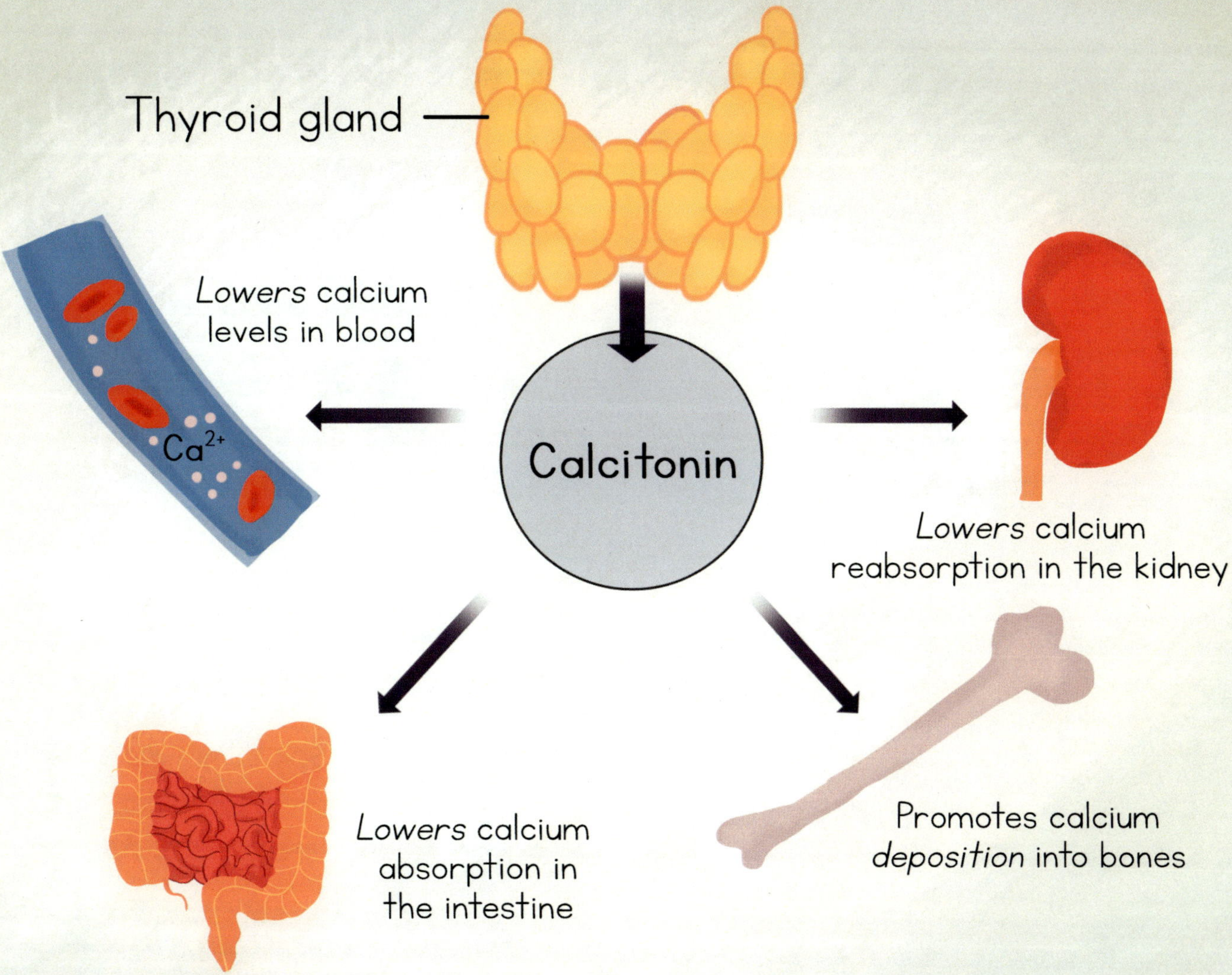

Calcitonin *lowers* the calcium level in our blood when it rises above the normal range.

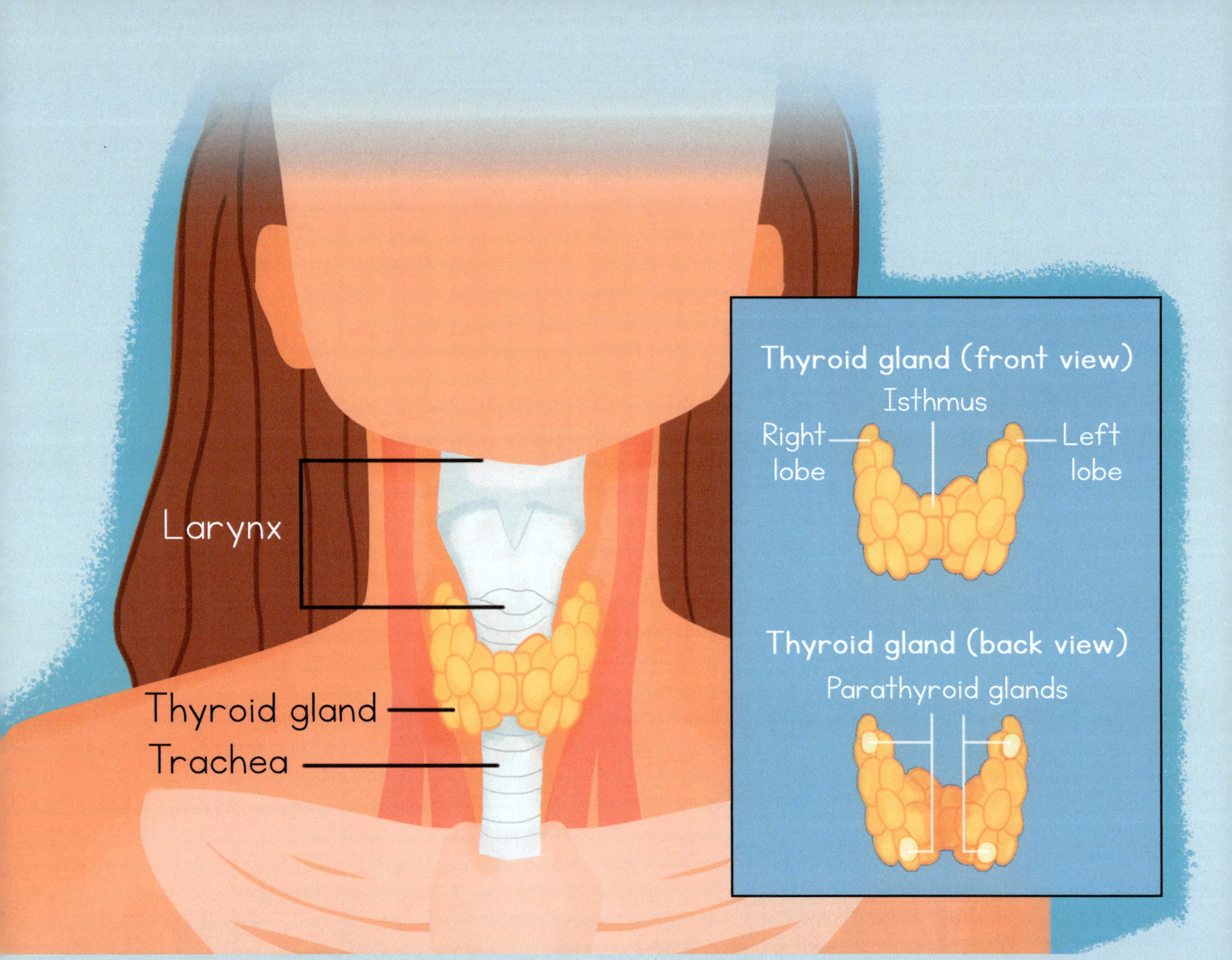

Behind the thyroid are four **parathyroid glands** that produce **parathyroid hormone (PTH)**.

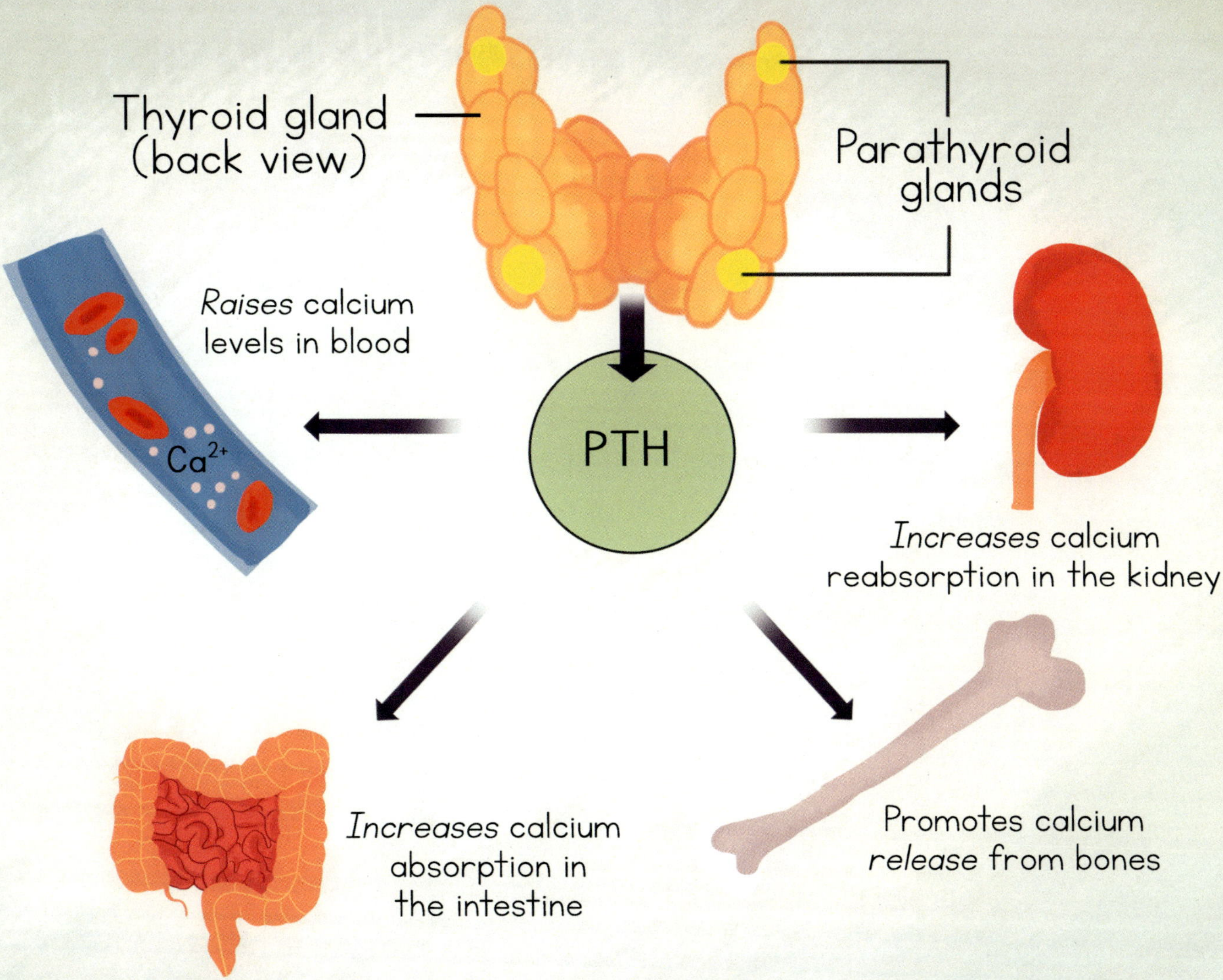

PTH *raises* the calcium level in our blood when it falls below the normal range.

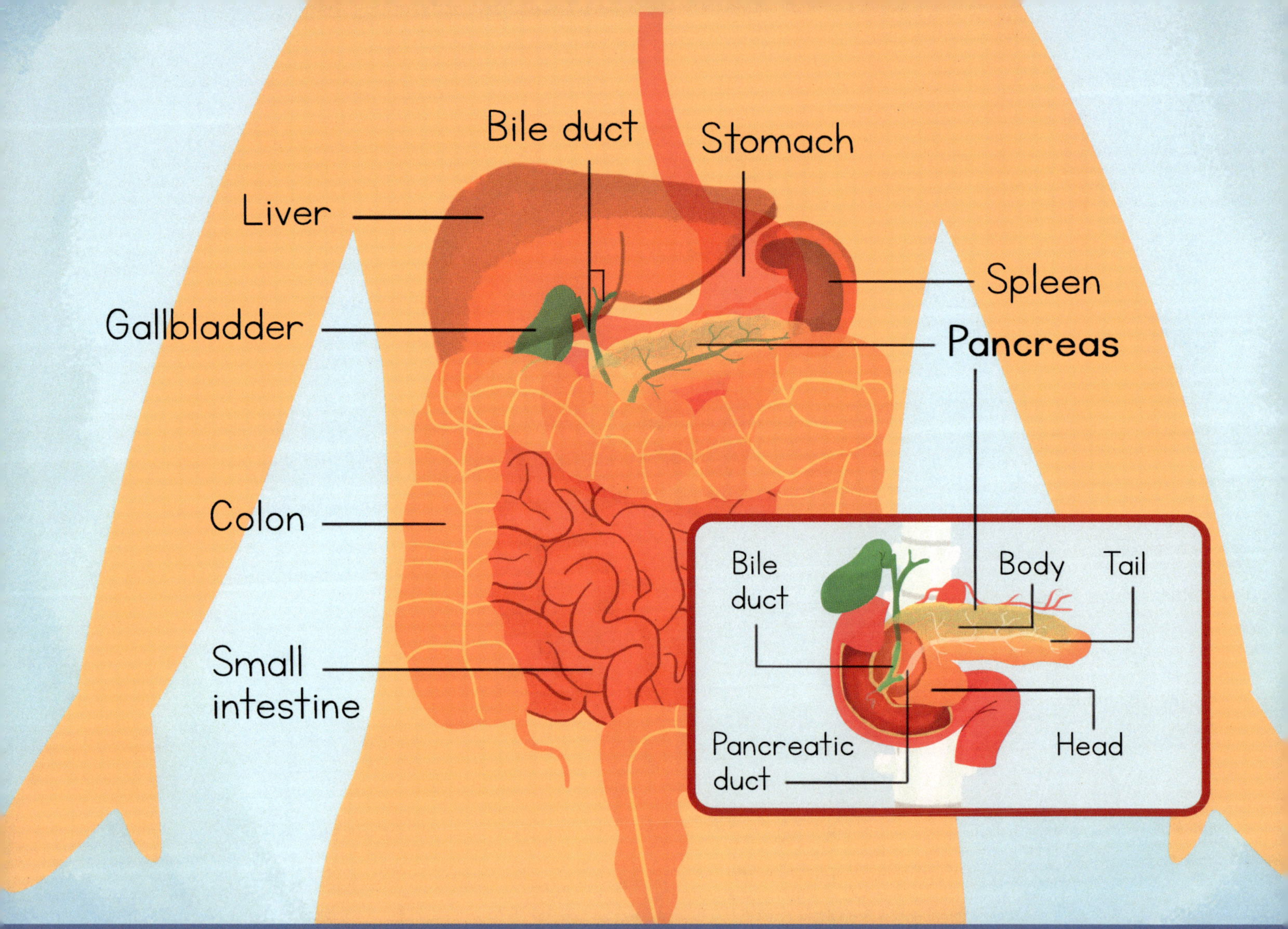

The **pancreas** is an organ in our belly between the stomach and spine. It produces two hormones called **insulin** and **glucagon**.

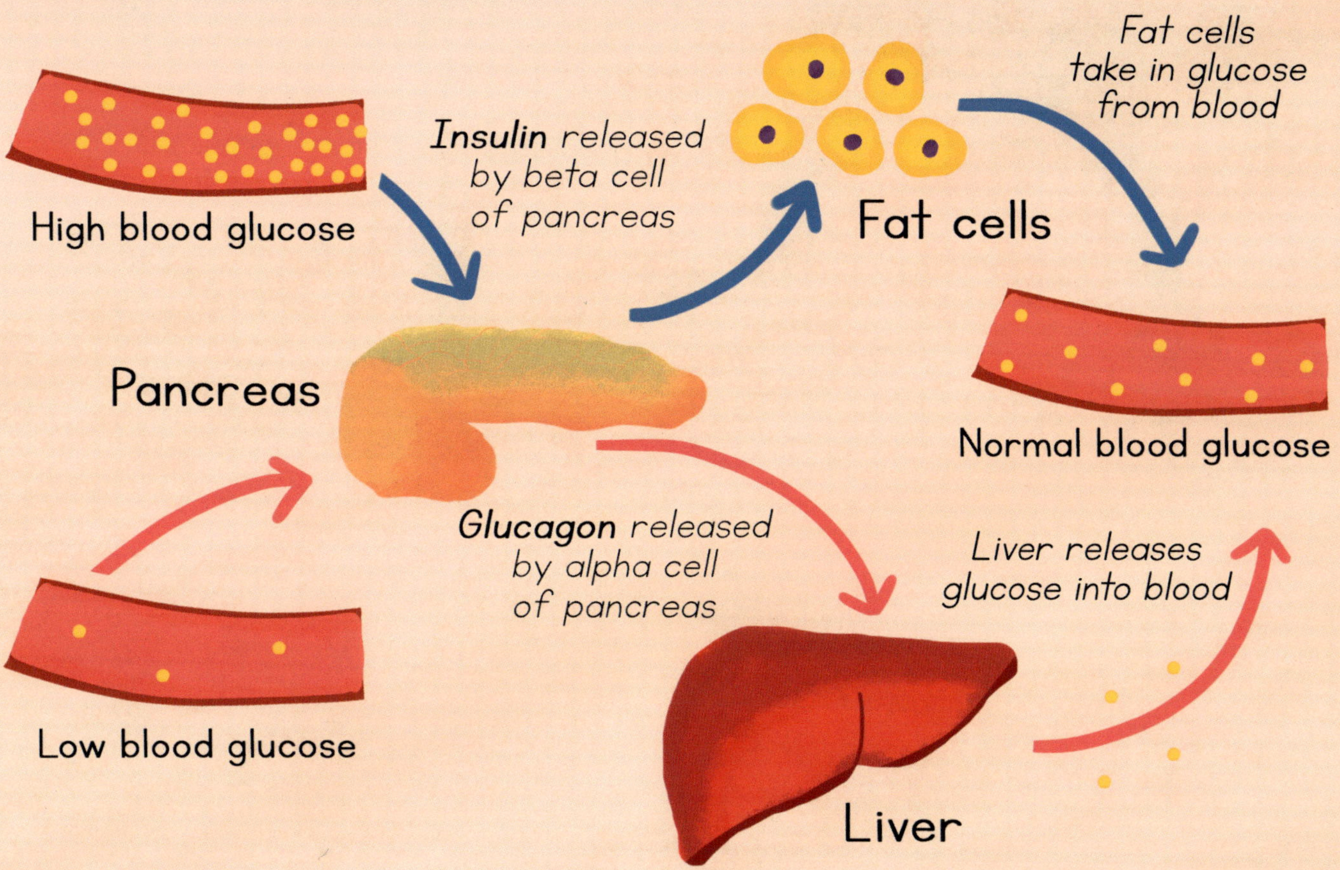

When your blood sugar levels are too high or too low, the pancreas releases **insulin** or **glucagon** to normalize blood sugar levels.

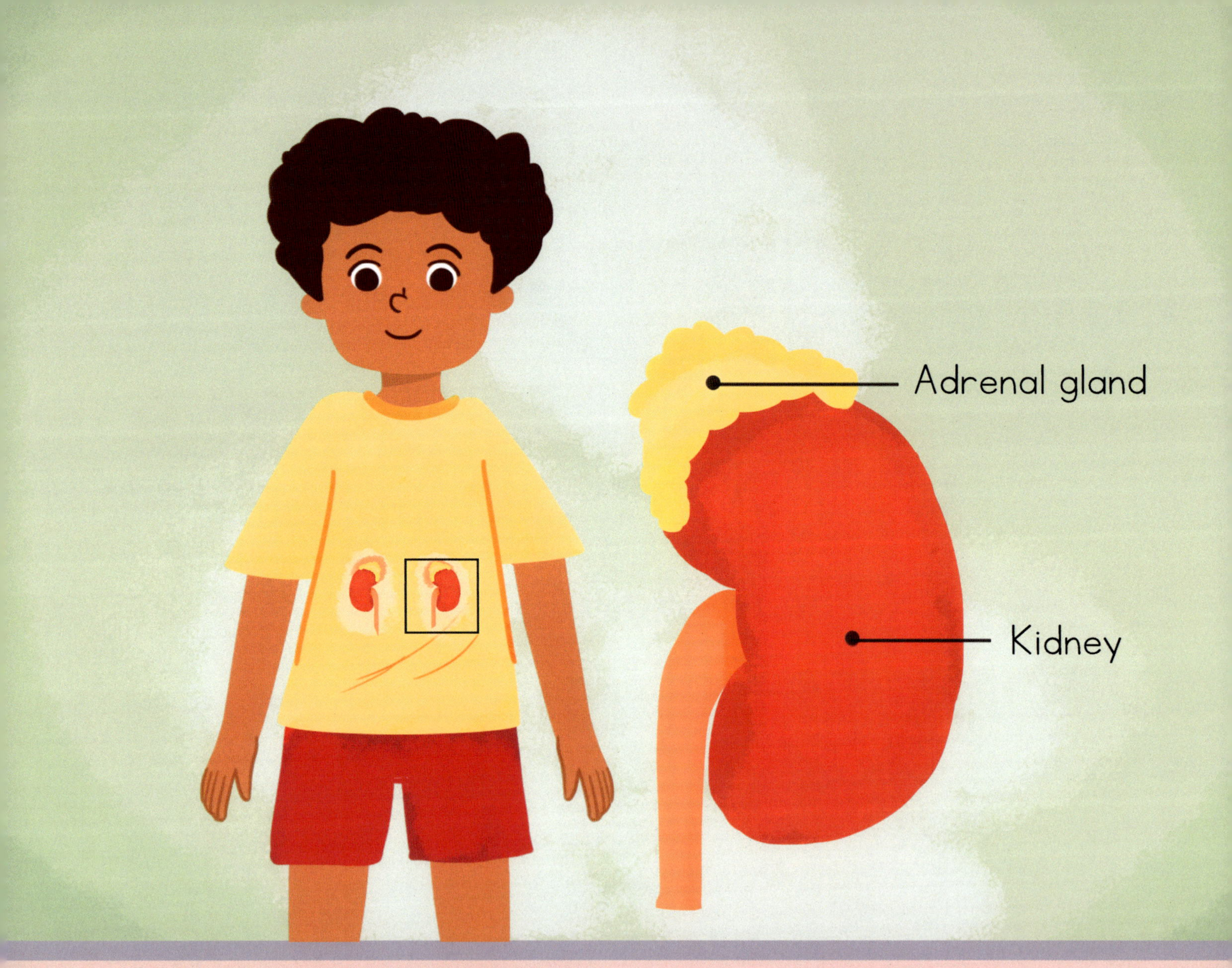

The **adrenal glands** are two small triangular organs that sit on top of each kidney.

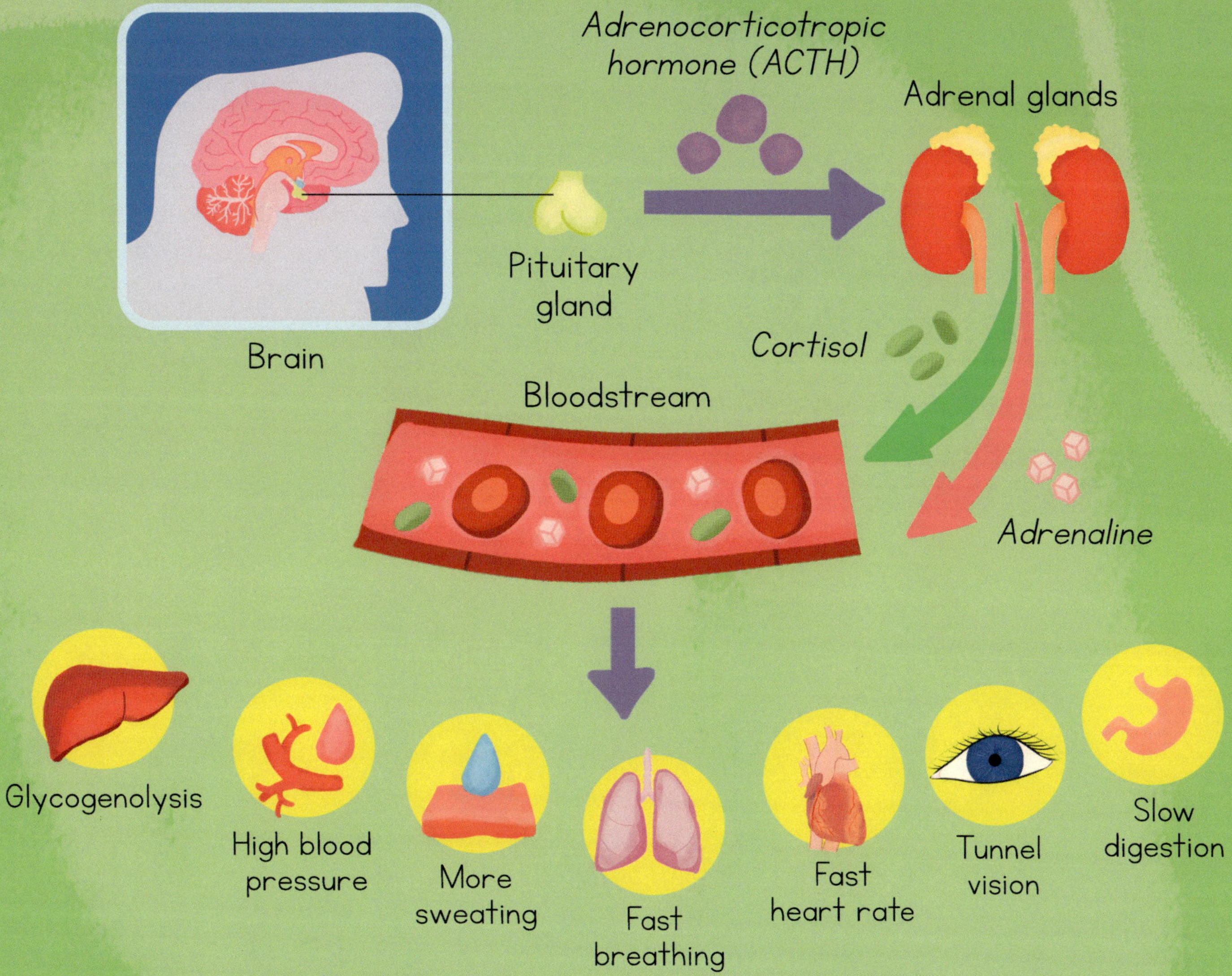

The adrenal glands produce stress hormones, such as **adrenaline** and **cortisol**, when our body is sick or under stress.

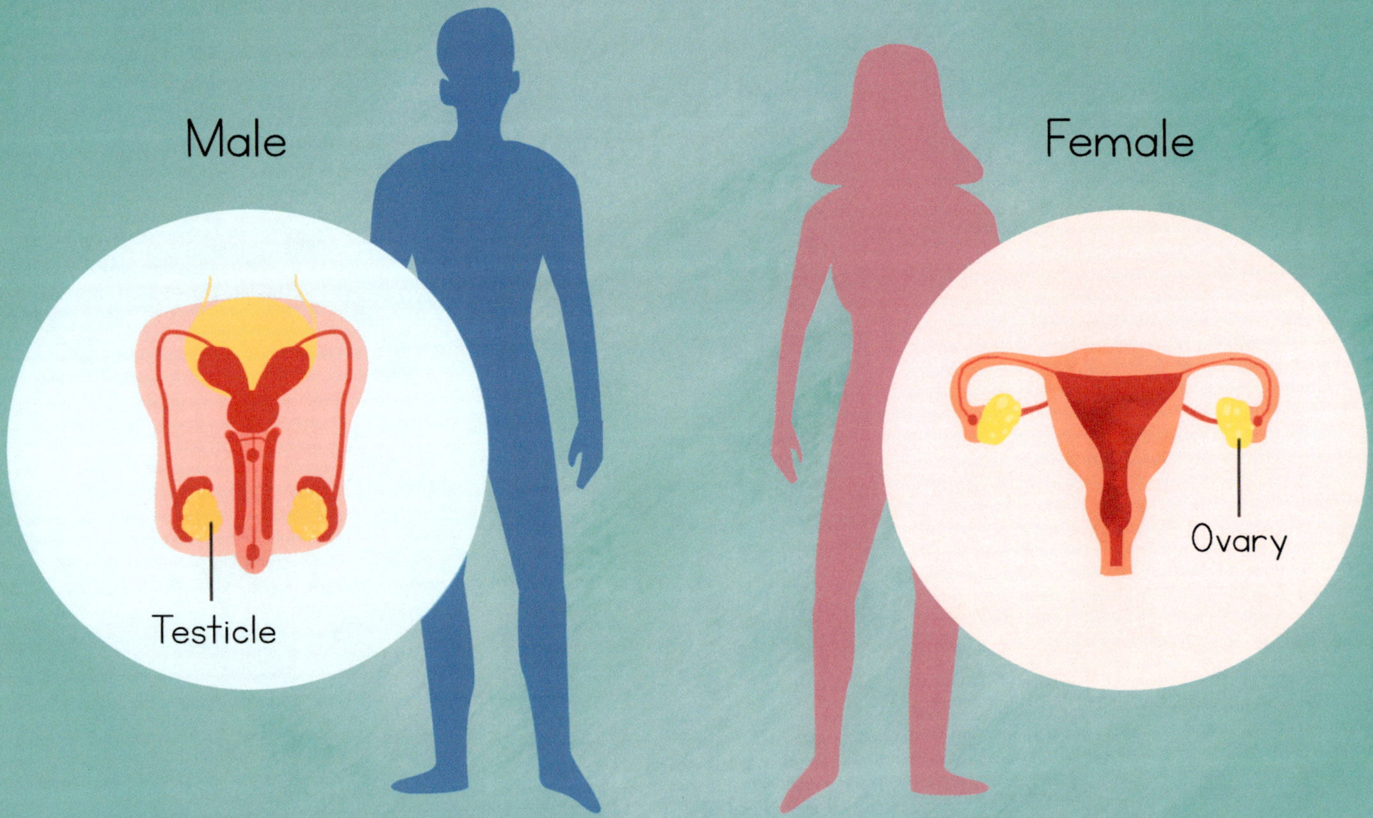

Gonads are our reproductive organs. Male gonads are called **testicles**, and female gonads are called **ovaries**.

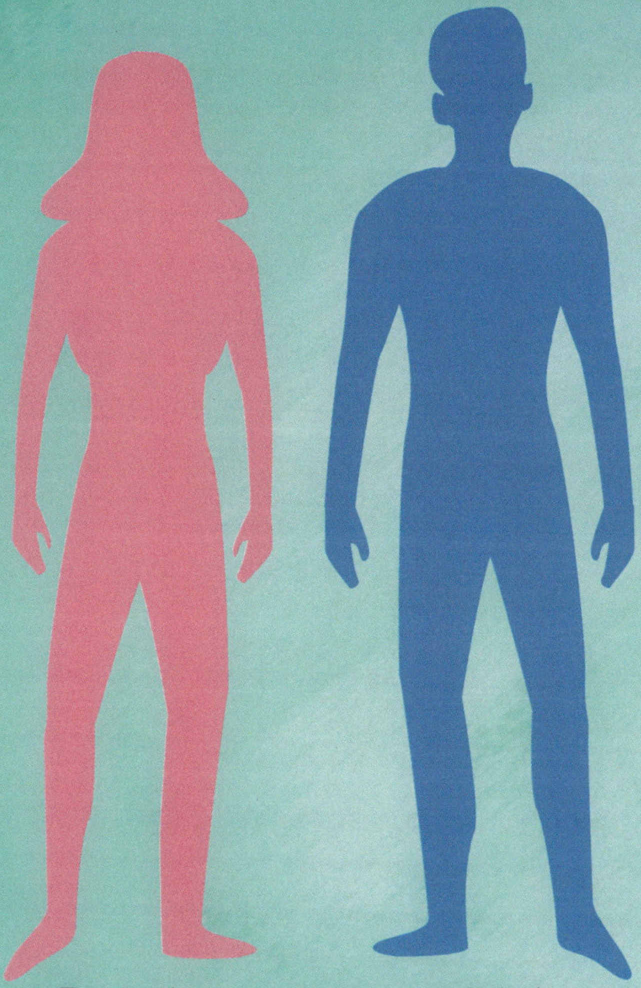

Female Male

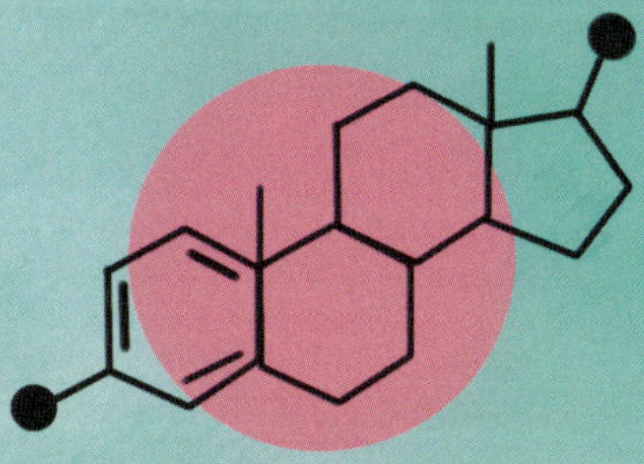

Estrogen

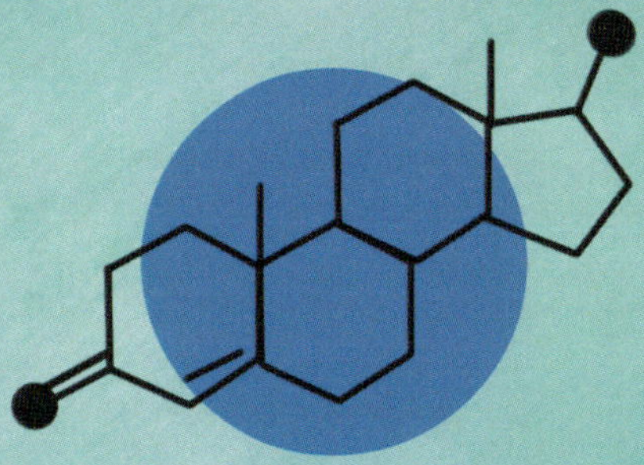

Testosterone

In males, testes make a hormone called **testosterone**. In females, ovaries make a hormone called **estrogen**.

Symptoms of hormonal imbalances

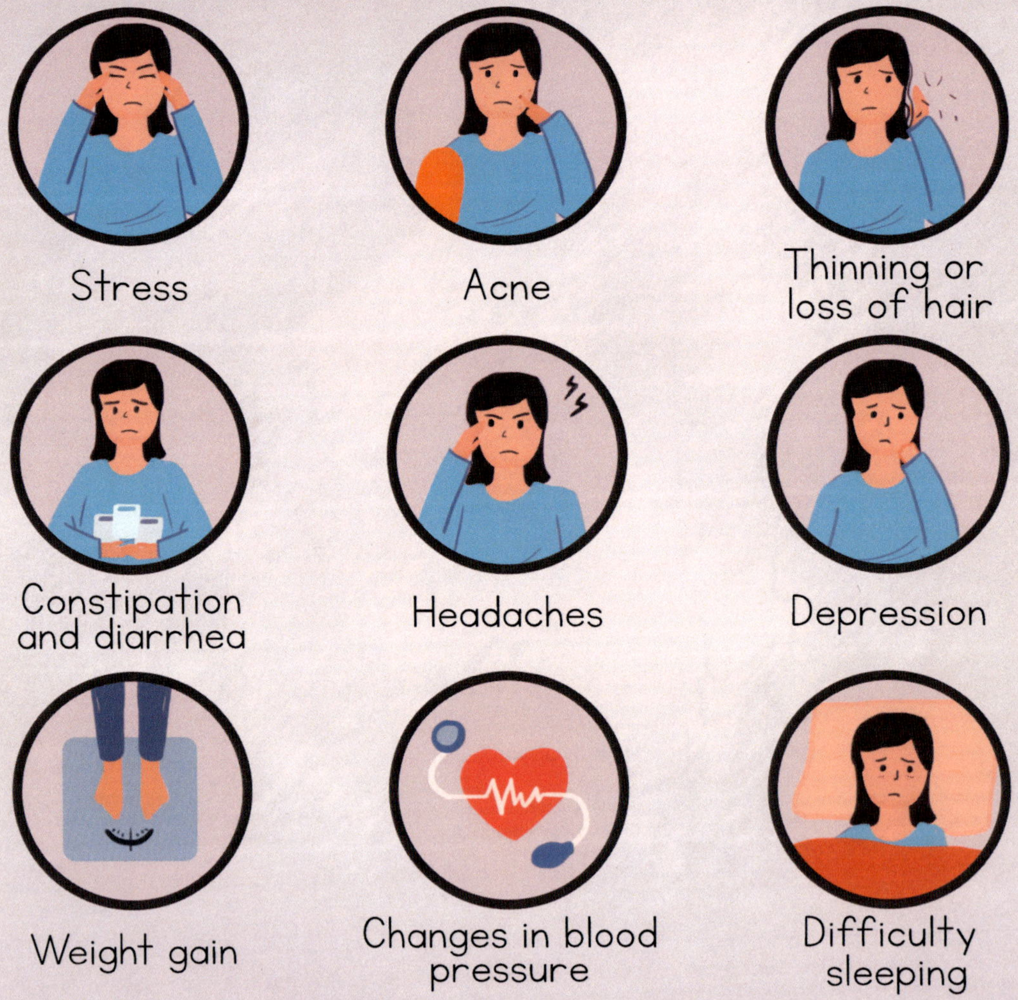

If problems with endocrine glands change our hormone levels, we might feel sick.

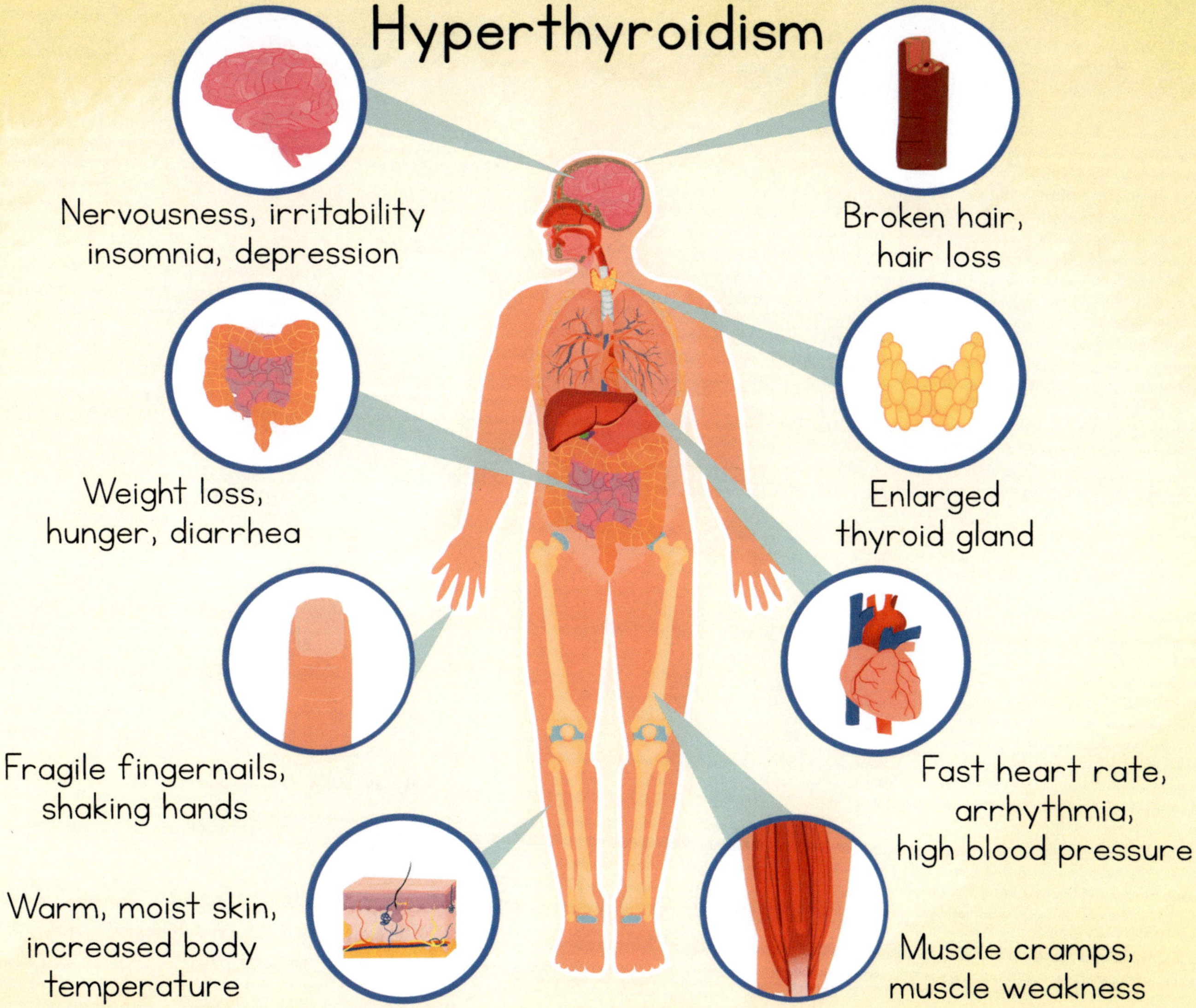

Patients with too *much* thyroid hormone might have weight loss, fast heart rate, anxiety, and diarrhea. This is called **hyperthyroidism**.

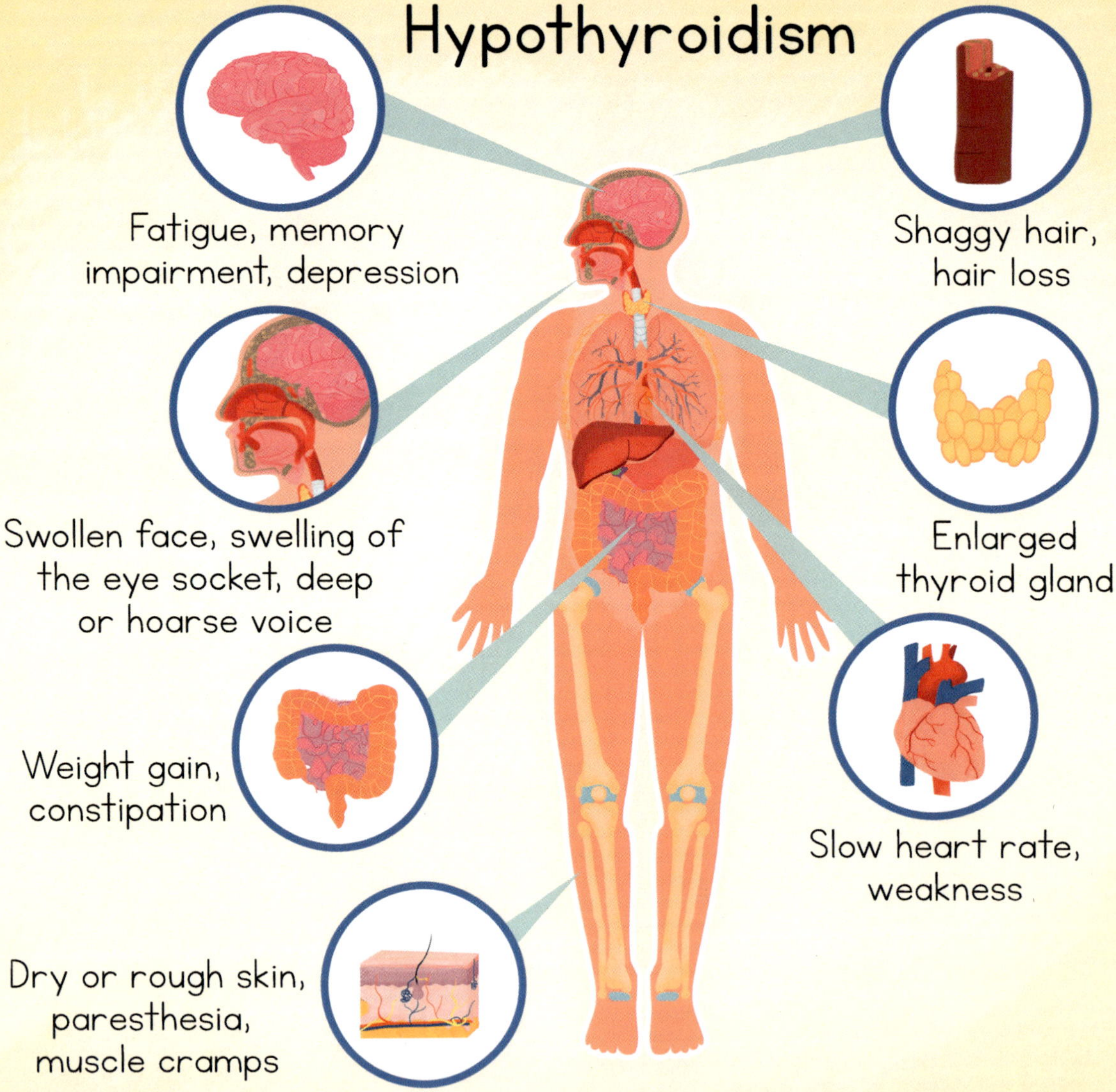

Patients with too *little* thyroid hormone might have weight gain, slow heart rate, depression, and constipation. This is called **hypothyroidism**.

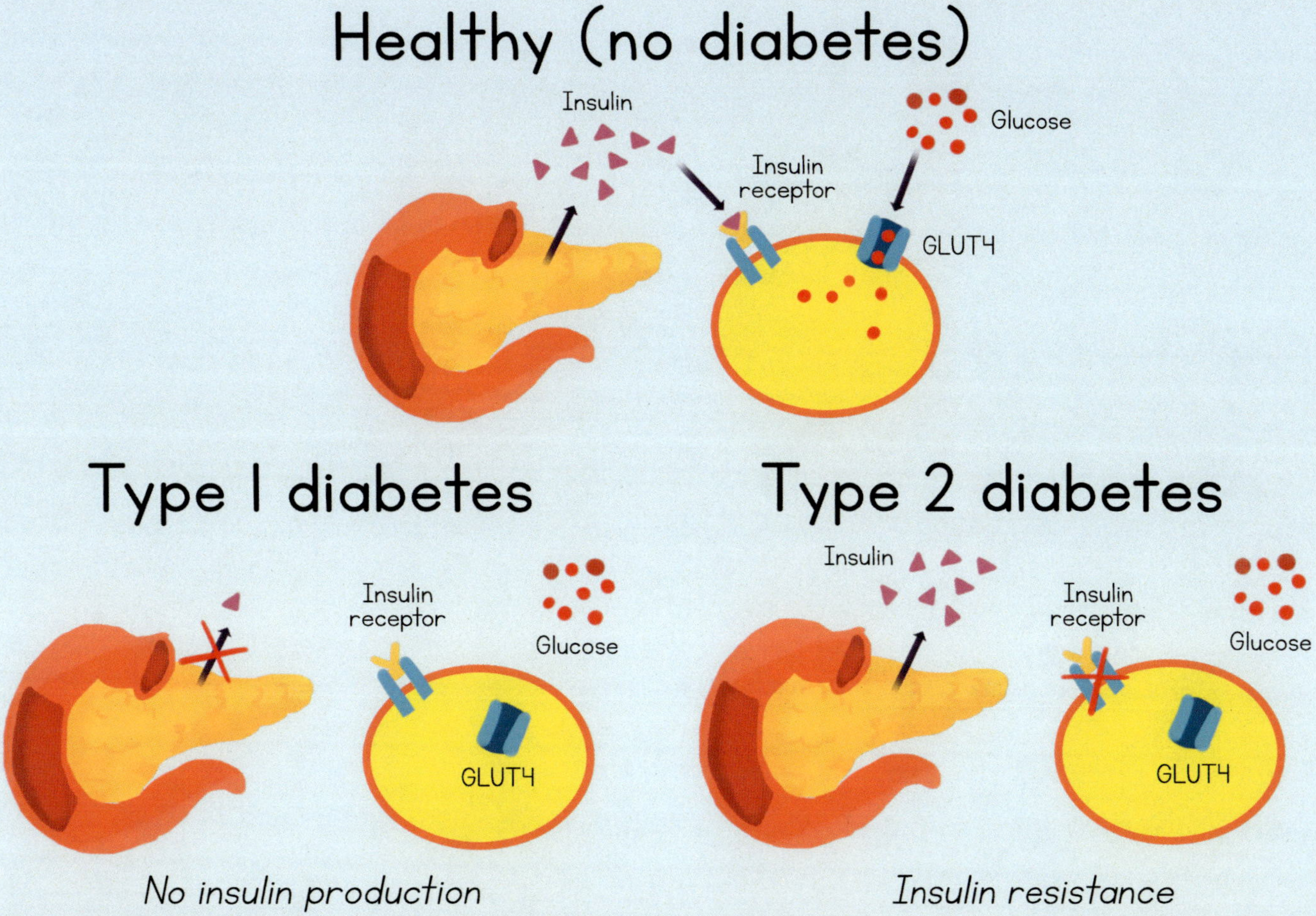

Diabetes mellitus is a condition where the body cannot make or respond to insulin normally. This causes high blood sugar levels and can make us thirsty and pee a lot.

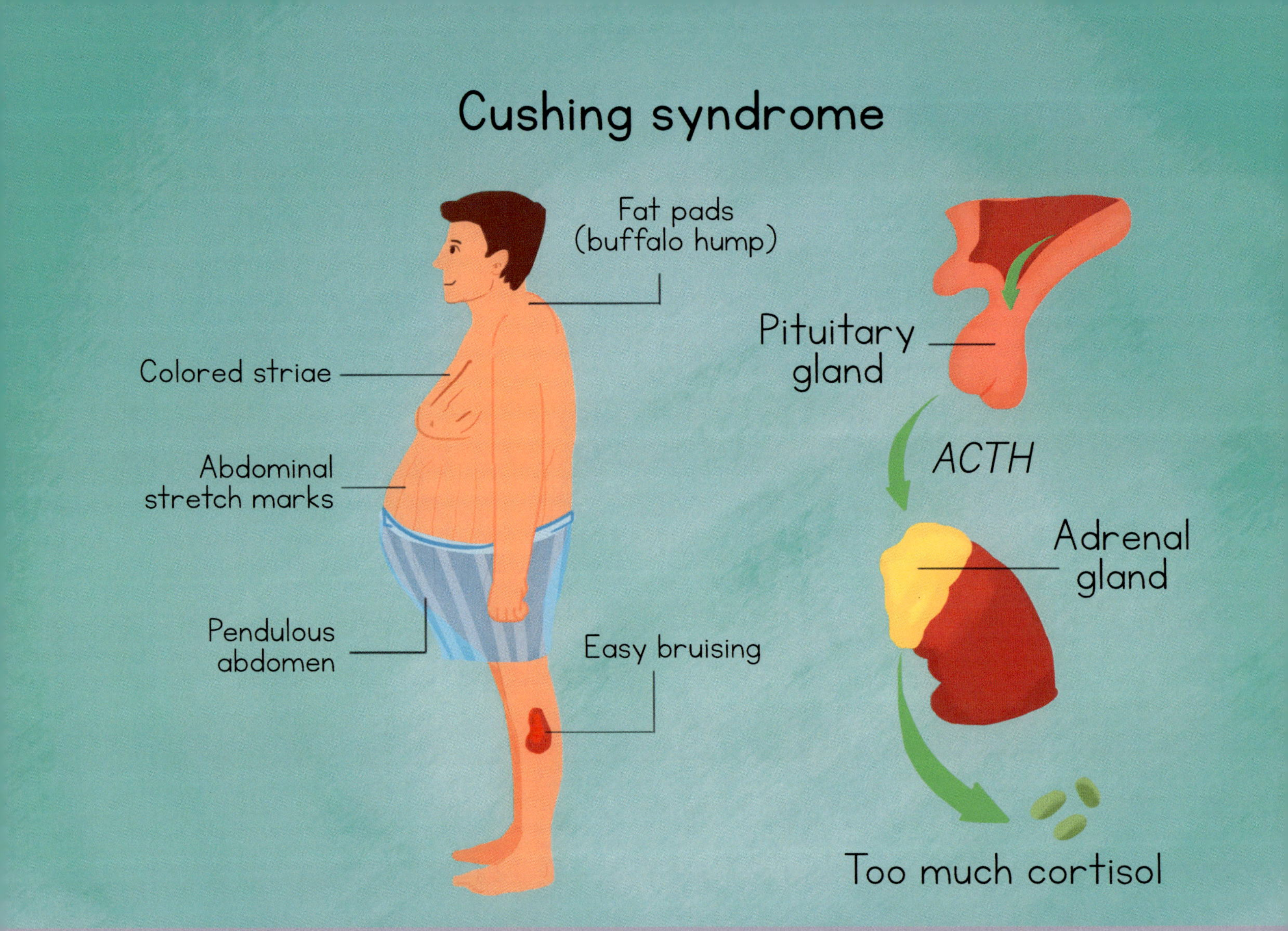

Cushing syndrome is a condition where the adrenal gland makes too much **cortisol**. This can cause muscle loss, weight gain, and easy bruising.

Pheochromocytoma

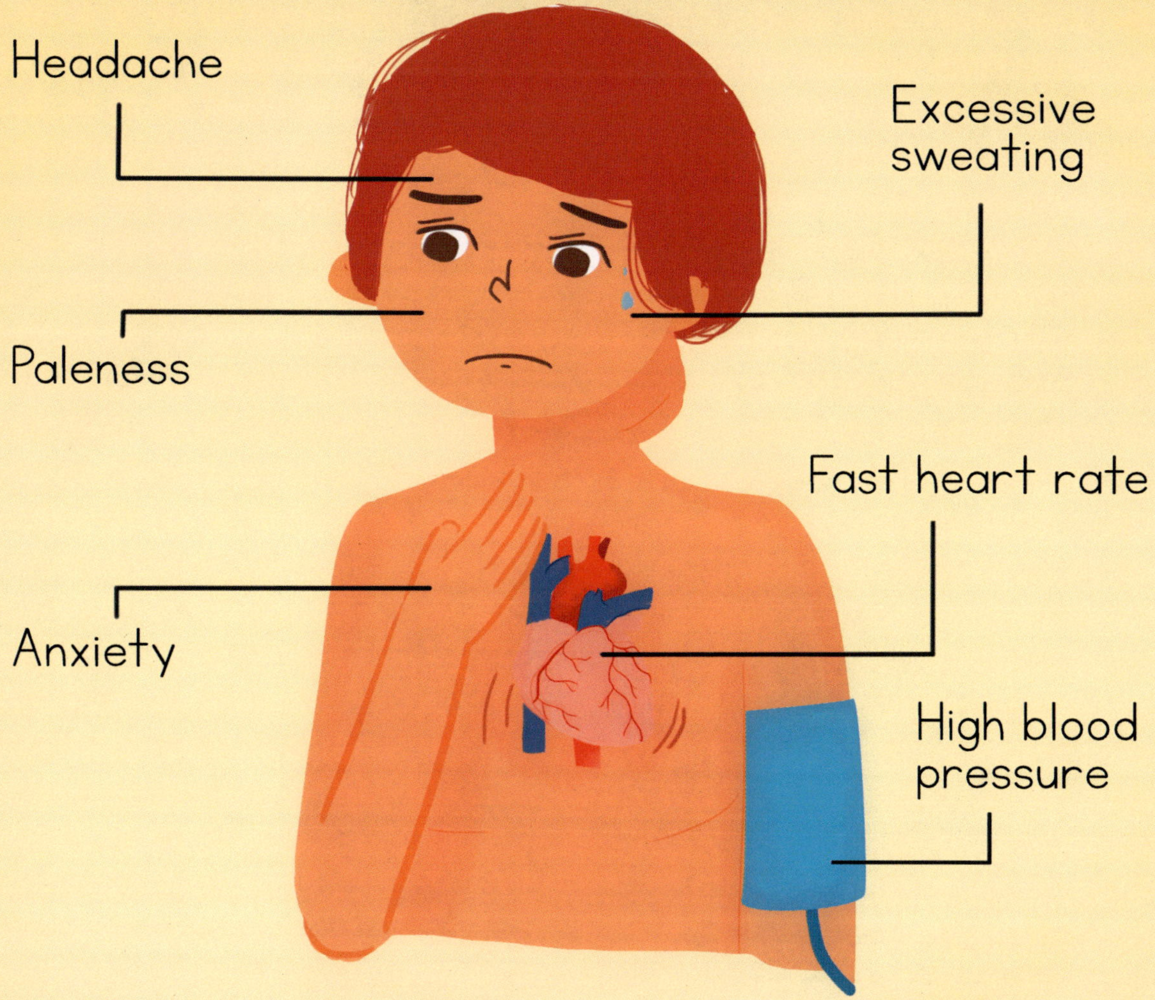

Pheochromocytoma is a condition where the adrenal glands make too much **adrenaline**, causing symptoms such as fast heart rate.

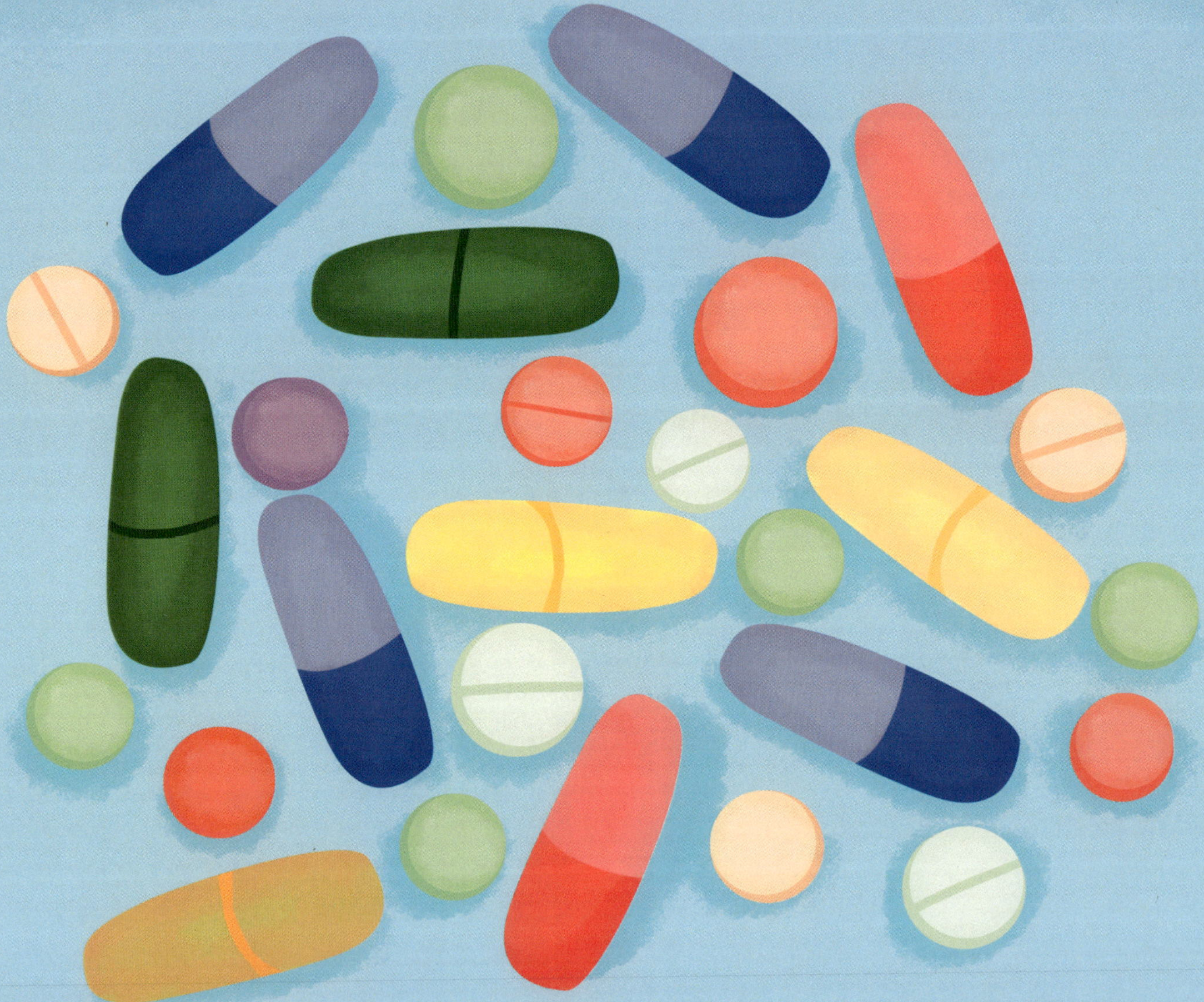

Patients with endocrine conditions might take medications that either increase or decrease the activity of certain hormones in their bodies.

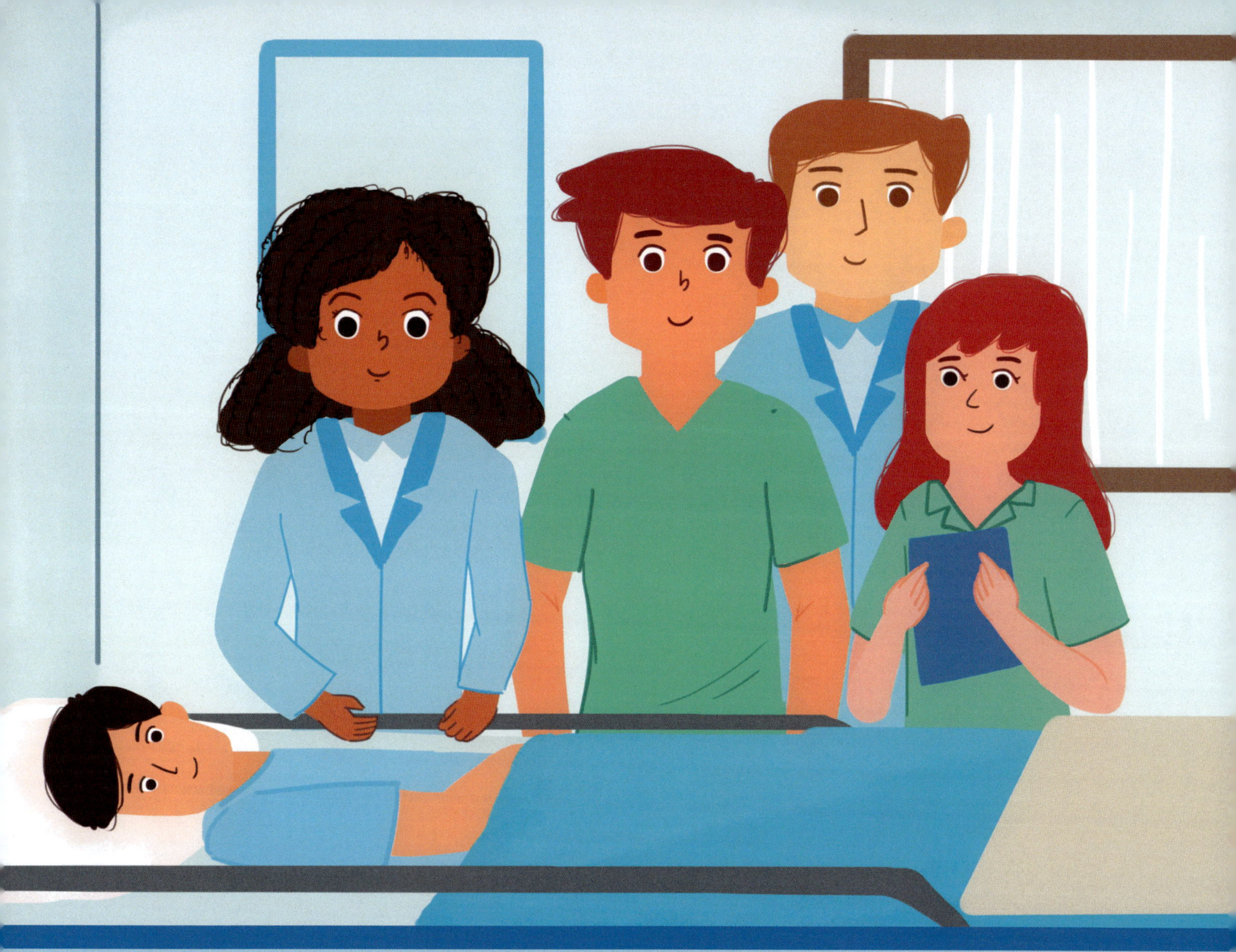

Fortunately, endocrinologists can diagnose and treat endocrine conditions by measuring and correcting hormone levels in the blood.

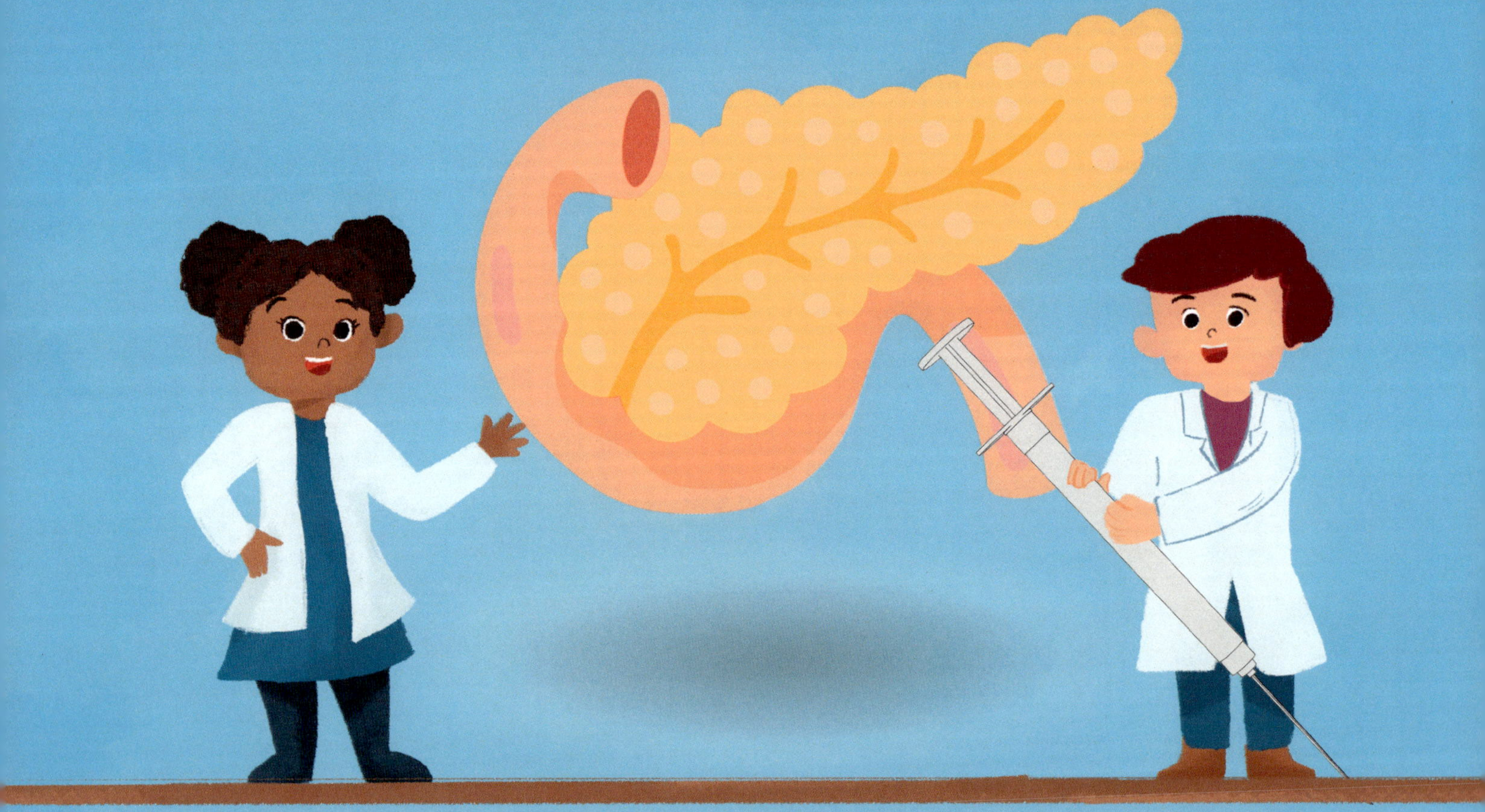

YOU'RE A FUTURE ENDOCRINOLOGIST!

Glossary

Cells (sel): basic building blocks of all living things

Hormone (HOR-mown): chemical made by our body that travels through our bloodstream to send messages to our cells

Endocrine glands: organs that make hormones released into the bloodstream

Pineal gland (PI-nee-uhl): pea-sized gland in our brain that produces melatonin

Pituitary gland (puh-TOO-uh-teh-ree): pea-sized gland in our brain that makes hormones, such as **ACTH**, **FSH**, **GH**, **LH**, **TSH**, and **PRL**, that control the activity of other organs and glands

Thyroid gland (THAI-royd): butterfly-shaped gland in our neck that produces thyroid hormone (called **T3** and **T4**) and **calcitonin**

Parathyroid glands (phe-ruh-THAI-royd): four pea-sized glands found on the back surface of the thyroid that produce **parathyroid hormone (PTH)**

Pancreas (PANG-kree-uhs): organ in our belly that makes **insulin** and **glucagon**

Adrenal glands (uh-DREE-nuhl): two small triangular organs that sit on top of each kidney; produce **adrenaline** and **cortisol**

Gonads (GOW-nadz): reproductive organs (**testes** in males, **ovaries** in females)

Hyperthyroidism: condition caused by too *much* thyroid hormone

Hypothyroidism: condition caused by too *little* thyroid hormone

Diabetes mellitus: condition where the body cannot make or respond to insulin

Cushing syndrome: condition where adrenal glands make too much **cortisol**

Pheochromocytoma (fee-oh-krow-moh-sai-TOW-mah): condition where the adrenal glands make too much **adrenaline**

Let's review what you learned!

1. What are the basic building blocks of all living things called?
2. What are the chemicals made by our body that travel through our bloodstream to send messages to our cells called? Where are they made?
3. Melatonin is produced by which endocrine gland? What is its role?
4. Which endocrine gland produces hormones that control the activity of other organs and glands? What are examples of these hormones produced?
5. Which hormone made by the pituitary gland helps you grow strong a tall?
6. Which hormone made by the pituitary gland controls thyroid gland activity?
7. Which hormones does the thyroid gland make, and what are their roles?
8. What are the four endocrine glands behind the thyroid called?
9. Which hormone does the parathyroid gland produce, and what is its role?
10. Which organ produces insulin and glucagon? What is each hormone's role?
11. Which endocrine glands are two small triangular organs that sit on top of each kidney? What hormones do they make?
12. Which endocrine glands are our reproductive organs?
13. Patients with too much or too little thyroid hormone have what conditions?
14. Patients who can't make or respond to insulin normally have what condition?
15. Patients who make too much cortisol or adrenaline have what conditions?

Medical School FOR KIDS™

Your Answers

1. ______________________________
2. ______________________________
3. ______________________________
4. ______________________________
5. ______________________________
6. ______________________________
7. ______________________________
8. ______________________________
9. ______________________________
10. ______________________________
11. ______________________________
12. ______________________________
13. ______________________________
14. ______________________________
15. ______________________________

Medical School FOR KIDS™

Answer Key

1. Cells
2. Hormones; endocrine glands
3. Pineal gland; makes us sleepy when it's time to go to bed
4. Pituitary gland; ACTH, endorphins, FSH, GH, LH, prolactin, TSH
5. Growth hormone (GH)
6. Thyroid-stimulating hormone (TSH)
7. Thyroid hormone (T3 and T4), which controls how fast our cells burn fuels from food to make energy; calcitonin, which lowers the calcium level in our blood when it rises above the normal range
8. Parathyroid glands
9. Parathyroid hormone; raises the calcium level in our blood when it falls below the normal range
10. Pancreas; insulin lowers blood sugar levels, glucagon raises blood sugar levels
11. Adrenal glands; cortisol and adrenaline
12. Gonads (testicles in males, ovaries in females)
13. Too much = hyperthyroidism; too little = hypothyroidism
14. Diabetes mellitus; Type 1 = can't make insulin, Type 2 = can't respond to insulin
15. Cortisol = Cushing syndrome; adrenaline = pheochromocytoma

Medical School FOR KIDS™

About the Authors

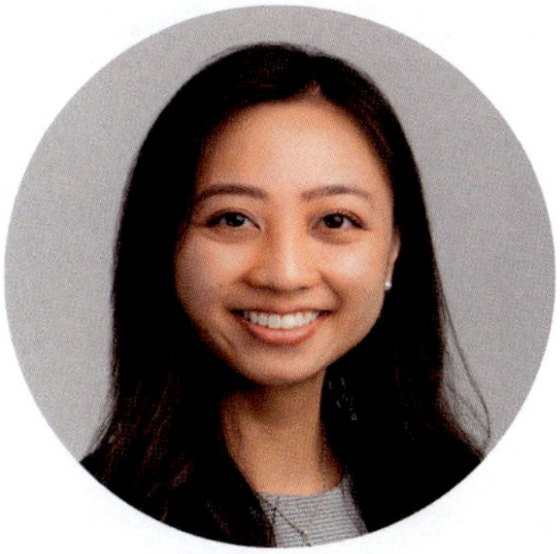

Betty Nguyen

Betty Nguyen was born in California but spent much of her childhood in Georgia, where she grew up on a chicken farm. She received a bachelor's degree in Biology from UCLA, where she received a full-ride Gates Millennium Scholarship through the Bill & Melinda Gates Foundation. Betty also received a full-tuition scholarship to attend medical school at the University of California, Riverside. Outside of work, Betty is a certified yoga instructor and licensed scuba diver. She also enjoys journalistic writing, cycling, and walking her two dogs in her free time.

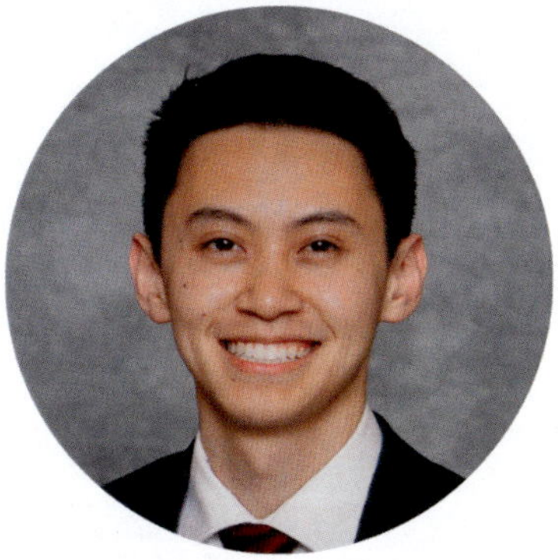

Brandon Pham

Brandon Pham was born and raised in California. He received a bachelor's degree in Microbiology, Immunology, and Molecular Genetics from UCLA, where he was a national Goldwater Scholar. He graduated from Stanford Medical School and is currently completing his residency in ophthalmology at the Bascom Palmer Eye Institute in Miami, Florida. Brandon spent many years teaching for several national test-preparation companies and is passionate about medical education for students of all ages. In his free time, Brandon enjoys traveling, playing tennis, and distance running.

Check out the rest of the books in our series!

Website: mdforkids.org

Instagram: @md.for.kids

Medical School FOR KIDS™

Made in the USA
Coppell, TX
12 November 2026

11803125R00024